Research Methods in Psychiatry

A Beginner's Guide

UNIVERS

Edited by
CHRIS FREEMAN
PETER TYRER

Research Methods in Psychiatry

A Beginner's Guide

GASKELL

©The Royal College of Psychiatrists 1989

ISBN 0 902241 29 X

Gaskell is an imprint of the Royal College of Psychiatrists,
17 Belgrave Square, London SW1

Distributed in North America
by American Psychiatric Press, Inc.

Phototypeset by Dobbie Typesetting Limited, Plymouth, Devon
Printed in Great Britain at the Alden Press, Oxford

Contents

List of contributors

Simon Backett, Senior Registrar, Medical Research Council Unit for Epidemiological Studies in Psychiatry, University Department of Psychiatry, Royal Edinburgh Hospital, Edinburgh EH10 5HF

Brian Ferguson, Consultant Psychiatrist, Research Office, Mapperley Hospital, Nottingham NG3 6AA

Chris Freeman, Consultant Psychotherapist, Senior Lecturer in Psychiatry, University of Edinburgh, Edinburgh EH10 5HF

Keith Hawton, Consultant Psychiatrist and Clinical Lecturer, Warneford Hospital and University Department of Psychiatry, Oxford OX3 7JX

Eve Johnstone, Honorary Consultant Psychiatrist, Northwick Park Hospital and Clinical Research Centre, Middlesex HA1 3UJ

Tony Johnson, Statistician, Medical Research Council Biostatistics Unit, Cambridge CB2 2BW

M. Timothy Lambert, Lecturer in Psychiatry, Academic Department of Psychiatry, St Mary's Hospital, London W2

Frank Margison, Consultant Psychotherapist, Gaskell House, Manchester M13 0EU

Graeme McGrath, Consultant Psychiatrist, Manchester Royal Infirmary, Manchester M13 9BX

Stephen Morley, Senior Lecturer in Clinical Psychology, Department of Psychiatry, University of Leeds, Leeds LS2 9JT

Siobhan Murphy, Senior Registrar in Psychiatry, St George's Hospital and Medical School, London SW17 0QT

David Peck, Area Clinical Psychologist, Clinical Psychology Service, Craig Dunain Hospital, Inverness IV3 6JU

Andrew Robinson, Honorary Senior Registrar, Medical Research Council Unit for Epidemiological Studies in Psychiatry, University Department of Psychiatry, Royal Edinburgh Hospital, Edinburgh EH10 5HF

Philip Snaith, Senior Lecturer in Psychiatry, Department of Clinical Science, St James' University Hospital, Leeds LS9 7TF

Peter Tyrer, Senior Lecturer in Psychiatry, St Charles' Hospital, London W10 6DZ

Preface

CHRIS FREEMAN and PETER TYRER

For the past three years we have been running regular two- and three-day research methodology courses for psychiatric trainees. These courses have demonstrated the need for a basic text on research methodology that is sensitive to the aims and resources available to trainees and that is suitable for someone starting out on their first research project. We have found considerable enthusiasm for psychiatric research among junior psychiatrists and an impressive array of original and clinically relevant research ideas. Why then is there not more research carried out by psychiatric trainees? Firstly, an enthusiastic trainee needs an enthusiastic and knowledgeable supervisor and such an individual seems to be hard for many trainees to find. Secondly, it is difficult for those of us working in university centres with easy access to research facilities to appreciate the difficulties that some trainees have. For example, on a recent course we had one trainee who had a four-hour round trip to visit a psychiatric library. Thirdly, trainees have many competing demands, such as the Membership Examination, night duty, etc., and many projects appear to get started but never completed, or completed and the results never analysed and written up.

We hope that this book will be helpful at all stages of a research project, although it can never be a substitute for good supervision. Many of the chapters are written by psychiatrists who have acted as tutors on our research methodology courses and most of them have been involved in supervising trainees in their own training schemes. We feel confident, therefore, that they have written in a way that is accessible and understandable to trainees.

We have included extensive sections in the book on rating scales and again this reflects our experience both in individual supervision and from running courses. Some of the most frequently asked questions concern what is an appropriate scale to use, how to find the reference for it, and how long it will take to administer. We have not included sections on statistics. We feel that there are numerous small statistics books available that cover all the main statistical tests that are likely to be needed. We have emphasised in the book that consulting a medical statistician is important and that it is useful to do that before starting research, not once the results have been collected.

We hope then that this book will help trainees to get started, help them avoid many of the pitfalls that frequently occur in planning and carrying out research, help maintain their enthusiasm and carry them through to their first published paper.

We wish those beginning research luck in what at times can appear futile, depressing, tedious, and repetitive. However, it can also be an exciting endeavour, and we hope very much that the balance remains on the positive attributes.

1 Getting started in research

CHRIS FREEMAN and PETER TYRER

Research recognises no boundaries of class, culture, or status. It is critical and iconoclastic, as indeed should be the psychiatric trainee. It is now recognised in most medical curricula that students should have some awareness of research methodology during their training, not because they should become research workers, but for the simple reason that an understanding of research and its principles is an aid to better clinical practice. The history of medicine is littered with examples of mistakes made as a consequence of slavish adherence to dogmatic assertion, and psychiatry, as a late-developing medical discipline, has recapitulated many of the same mistakes in its short history.

Psychiatric trainees, whatever their research aspirations, need to learn how to observe and be sensitive to the unexpected. Most of the major advances in medicine have been made by following up chance observations in a logical and consistent way. Jenner's observations of cowpox, Fleming's of penicillin and Bowlby's of childhood separation did not require intellectual genius; they depended on observation untrammelled by preconceptions. All doctors should be capable of this.

This chapter aims to give general guidelines to the trainee who would like to know how a research idea can be converted into an investigation that will yield a useful result. But no amount of knowledge of research methodology will necessarily create a good project. The value of any investigation depends on the question being asked. It is this that determines the originality and value of research rather than the mechanism whereby it is tested. It is therefore far better for the trainee to develop research notions or ideas which can then be shaped into testable hypotheses rather than rely on someone else's suggestions or a casual review of the literature. If a research project is worth doing and invitations to carry it out have already appeared in print, it is quite probable that the investigation is already underway. Investigators are much more likely to see their project through when they have developed hypotheses from their own observations.

The aim of your research

This is the most important part of any research endeavour and is obviously independent of methodology. A bad research idea will produce bad results no matter how good the methodology used to explore it. In selecting an issue that seems to be appropriate for research, the following questions need to be asked before beginning. If they are not answered before you start, a great deal of hard work could be wasted.

(a) Why do you want to do the research?

If the answer is only 'to get a publication for my curriculum vitae' the work is likely to fail. Research has to be of some value to others if it is worth doing at all. The need to publish is understandable in a competitive age but should not be the only motivation. Table 1.1 gives some other motives for research, along with their likely probability!

(b) If the work is worth doing, why hasn't it been done before?

Research workers sometimes bemoan that there are 'no good ideas left'. It is still common for research to be carried out on subjects that leads to interesting results but which, on perusal of the literature, turns out to have been published before. A good literature search is essential before starting any research project (see below). A replication study should be planned, not accidental (see below).

(c) What results do you expect from the research work?

This question needs to be answered for two important reasons. The first is that the results may be completely predictable before beginning the investigation and do not therefore contain the element of doubt which is

TABLE 1.1
Reasons for doing research

Reason	Predicted success probabilities!
Nobel prize	$P \leqslant 0.000001$
Knighthood	$P \leqslant 0.00001$
Fame, prestige, glory	$P \leqslant 0.0001$
Changing our views of the world	$P \leqslant 0.0001$
Getting published	$P = 0.1$
Helping pass exams by learning research methods	$P = 0.2$
Modifying practice (at least yours)	$P = 0.3$
Getting a better job	$P = 0.7$
Keeping a critical attitude	$P = 0.75$
Enjoyment (sometimes)	$P = 0.8$

essential to any research inquiry. For example, there is little point in carrying out an investigation to determine whether tall people weigh more than short people, even if there has been no previous study in the scientific literature. However, there are many well known beliefs that have not been formally tested (e.g. the effects of blood letting by leeches) and whose investigation might provide some valuable insight. The second reason is the important one of bias. It is an unfortunate fact that research workers tend to find the results they expected before they started their work, and it is worthwhile making a note of what your expectations are before you start. This may subsequently be disclosed in published work when the results are presented.

(d) What are the likely implications of your research, including both positive and negative findings?

Good research has significant implications whether the findings turn out to be positive or negative. A great deal of research, however, seems to be carried out because it is technically feasible and can be carried out in a short time, but which has little or no longer-term implications. The recent spate of investigations into the dexamethasone suppression test is a good example. Beware of this trap by asking this question. If there are no significant implications do not proceed.

(e) Do I need advice before I go any further?

Before starting any research project it is advisable to discuss it with others. Sometimes investigators are reluctant to do this because they do not like to share their new ideas with other people in case they are stolen from them. In practice this occurs seldom, and not usually at an early stage, and it is a good idea to discuss your general ideas with a colleague whom you both trust and respect before going any further. This will often save a great deal of trouble in the long term.

Reviewing the literature

The best starting point is a good review article, although often if the area you are researching is relatively novel this will not be available. The *Index Medicus* is a useful starting base, providing you are relatively economical with your key words. The same applies to the two most widely used medical computer searches, MEDLARS and MEDLINE. These are available in most university libraries although sometimes a small fee may have to be paid. Some of the key words in these two schemes are not particularly well suited to psychiatric literature searches; if possible try to discuss the topic you are researching with an experienced user to help pick the most appropriate key words to use. Another very useful literature source is PSY-LIT, which was relatively recently made available in the UK and covers a wide range of psychological journals, many of which are not covered by MEDLINE. It runs on a microcomputer and is very user-friendly. Because all the data are stored on disks which are updated every six months, there is no delay in getting your references, and if inappropriate key words are used which generate few or many thousands of citations, it is possible to alter them before getting a print out. PSY-LIT should be available in most university libraries.

Development of a hypothesis

In developing a hypothesis it is usually wise to follow the agnostic viewpoint of Carl Popper that science exists to disprove hypotheses rather than to prove them. Thus no hypothesis can said to be right; the best hypothesis is the closest approximation to the truth that we have at present, but there is always the possibility that it will be replaced by another at a later date. For this reason hypotheses that are tested in scientific research are usually null hypotheses. If a null hypothesis is disproved then it is reasonable to entertain the positive hypothesis until the next point of testing it.

Hypotheses have to be precisely formulated questions rather than vague statements, and much care is needed in preparing them. For example:

Vague hypothesis: 'Does psychotherapy help patients with anorexia nervosa?'

Precisely formulated hypothesis: 'Does psychotherapy in the form of cognitive therapy, when given for ten weeks, lead to a significantly greater gain in weight in anorectic patients than in those not receiving cognitive therapy?'

Null hypothesis: 'There is no difference in the weight gain of patients with anorexia nervosa when treated with cognitive therapy compared with a control procedure.'

The design features of a clinical study

The chapters that follow will deal with research designs in greater detail, but it may be helpful to ask yourself the following questions at intervals as you plan your project.

(a) Is the objective of the study clearly and sufficiently described?
(b) Are clear diagnostic criteria used?
(c) Can you give a clear statement about the source of subjects?
(d) Are you using concurrent controls rather than historical controls?
(e) Are the treatments well defined?
(f) Are you using random allocation, and if so, what type?
(g) Will the trial be blind, and if so, how will you ensure this?
(h) Do you have appropriate outcome measures?

(i) Using these measures, do you have defined criteria of outcome?

(j) Have you carried out a power calculation (Ch. 2) to help determine the most appropriate sample size?

Getting supervision

A good supervisor is essential for a trainee carrying out research. At times, research projects can be lonely and dispiriting, especially when subject recruitment grinds to a halt. Supervision does not necessarily need to be frequent, although you are particularly likely to need help and constructive criticism while planning the study and at the writing up stage. Most good supervisors are extremely busy and it is important to use your supervision time fruitfully. The following section, 'Keeping a research diary', may help you with this. It is important that you and your supervisor negotiate exactly what is to be done at each stage, and it is usually helpful for you to be given deadlines. Your supervisor does not necessarily need to be an expert in the field of your research. It is more important that he/she has a general appreciation of the research design and has a critical, inquiring attitude.

Keeping a research diary

When you start, it is useful to keep a notebook for that particular project. At the beginning you should plan out in as much detail as possible the course of the project, allowing time for the literature search, designing a protocol, submission to an ethics committee, recruitment of subjects, collection of data, etc. Also note in the diary as many of your own predictable life events (e.g. Christmas, revision and sitting of exams, annual holidays). Allow for these things in the planning of your research, and try to fit blocks of research around them. For example, plan what is going to happen to patients when you are on holiday, and remember that it is unlikely you will be able to recruit new subjects or get people to attend for follow-up around Christmas and New Year. Allow too for the fact that if you are in training you may have to move from post to post. Thus at the beginning of your diary there should be a detailed plan of all the stages of research mapped out month by month and related to other events in your life. An example is given in Fig. 1.1.

As the research progresses you should use the notebook to record all important decisions that you make: it can be very frustrating to reach the end of a research project and have no idea why you decided to alter a particular facet of the research or why a particular subject was excluded. Also write down all interesting anecdotes which occur as you go through the project. You will find that if you have a relatively complete research notebook, analysis of data and writing up will be much less of a task.

Date	Main stages of study	Study tasks	Life events
Oct. 88	Literature review	MEDLINE/PSY-LIT research	
Nov. 88			
Dec. 88	Initial protocol		Christmas holidays
Jan. 89	Pilot studies	Try questionnaire on individual patients	
Feb. 89	Submit to ethics committee		Revision
		Contact GPs and	
Mar. 89		consultants	Exams
April 89	Main study	Final draft of questionnaire ready	
May 89			
		Give to	
June 89		GP patients	
		Definite cases	
July 89		Borderline cases	Summer holiday
		Physically ill	
Aug. 89		Psychiatrically ill samples	New post in rotation
Sept. 89			
Oct. 89		Test–retest reliability study	Revision
Nov. 89			Exams
	Complete main		
Dec. 89	study	Code and check all data	
Jan. 90	Analysis		Rotation change of job
Feb. 90			
Mar. 90			Moving house
April 90	Writing up		
May 90			
June 90	Study ends		Present results at scientific meeting

Fig. 1.1   Typical research plan at the beginning of a research diary. The project was to design, pilot and validate a screening questionnaire for somatisation disorder in general practice

Designing a protocol

This is an important exercise, even if you are not applying for a grant. Most grant-giving bodies, such as the Medical Research Council, Wellcome Trust, and the Mental Health Foundation, require protocols to be submitted in a particular form. It is useful to have a look at these application forms, as they give helpful guidance as to how a protocol should be set out. The general steps required are listed below. Although you may be keen to get on with your project without going through this stage, it will save you time later and will be very helpful when you come to writing up, as your method section will be virtually written for you. It is best to start off with a first draft that is overinclusive, trying to put down in rough form as many ideas and alternative trial designs as possible, and then to discuss them with your supervisor.

The procotol: steps in planning a study

(a) Getting an idea

(b) General background reading and the more formal literature search
(c) Form a specific aim (hypothesis of study)
(d) Design a study protocol to attempt to falsify this hypothesis. This should include the following:
    (i) patient selection criteria
    (ii) treatment schedules
    (iii) methods of patient evaluation
    (iv) study design
    (v) how subjects will be randomised
    (vi) patient consent
    (vii) size of study
    (viii) monitoring of study progress
    (ix) forms and data handling
    (x) protocol deviations
    (xi) statistical analysis
    (xii) plans for administration/staff and finance
(e) Apply for ethical approval
(f) Run a pilot study
(g) Redesign study, if necessary (different sample size, rate of recruitment)
(h) Contact ethics committee and inform them of changes
(i) Run main experiment
(j) Collect and analyse data
(k) Publish so as to inform and allow for replication.

Applying to an ethics committee

You will almost certainly have to do this for any research that you carry out. Again the process differs from committee to committee, but the list below gives some of the questions that ethics committees need to know.

What is the object of the study (explained in terms appropriate to the intelligent layman)?

In what way will this study either advance medical knowledge or benefit the individual patient?

Will subjects be in-patients, out-patients, GP patients or healthy volunteers?

How will subjects/patients be recruited (by advertisement, from GP referrals, successive out-patient attenders, etc.)?

What selection criteria will be used for subjects?

Has statistical advice been sought on the size and design of the project?

What procedures will be carried out on the subjects/patients?

What drug will be administered, if any?

What risks are there to subjects?

What discomfort will there be for subjects?

What information will be given to subjects?

How will informed consent be obtained, and will this be obtained from all subjects?

How will consent be recorded? (Many committees require a copy of the patient information sheet and consent form to be sent to them)

If the subject is a patient in a dependent relationship to the investigator, have you considered having an independent person explain the study and obtain consent, in accordance with the Declaration of Helsinki on the Ethics of Medical Research?

Will there be an interval between giving the information and obtaining consent?

Will subjects be informed of their right to withdraw?

What information will be given to subjects' GPs, if any?

Will payment be made to subjects, and if so is this just reimbursement of expenses or is a fee involved?

How is the study being funded? Is any payment or other form of reimbursement being made directly to any of the investigators?

What security precautions will be taken to safeguard the confidentiality of data on patients?

Some ethical issues in research

Subjects sometimes find research stressful. If drugs are given or physical procedures applied there may be discomfort, even the possibility of harm. If personal information is divulged to the researcher, harm may result to the subject if this information passes beyond the researcher. If a new treatment is being tested, there may be unknown side-effects or possibly even a poor outcome. On the other hand, a subject may benefit directly, sometimes greatly, if a new therapy is on trial. There may be benefit to future sufferers, or, more distantly, benefit to future research efforts if the research project is training experience for the researcher. Subjects invited to participate in research should be given a chance to weigh these possible benefits against the risk to them of stress or harm resulting from their participation.

To enable the subject to make a judgement he/she must be informed of:

(a) each of the types of harm that could result from participation

(b) the magnitude of the risk of each of these forms of harm

(c) the kinds of benefit that may follow from the research and the likelihood of these benefits

(d) whether they may benefit directly or whether the benefit may be for other or future sufferers from a given disorder.

Sometimes a study is poorly designed; for example, it may not be able to answer the question it poses for a logical reason, or because the sample is poorly chosen or so small as to yield a result which could quite likely have occurred by chance. In such instances, the subject may tacitly assume he/she is contributing to advances in medical knowledge when in fact a design fault precludes the study from producing a useful result. The committee may consider such research unethical.

Getting subjects

One of the biggest problems in research is finding a sufficient number of subjects. Obviously this is less of a problem with retrospective case studies, also called 'archival research'. Here the subjects have already been identified and one does not have to rely on new recruitment. Even in these circumstances it can be surprising how large the wastage is from a subject list. A computer print-out from a case register of patients all of a single diagnosis may reveal some who have been misdiagnosed, and a few patients whose case notes do not seem to exist at all; there may be a whole string of other reasons why your previously clear-cut group of patients has to be whittled to a smaller sample. This is before one begins to tackle the fact that some patients will have died and many may have moved away.

When one comes to prospective research, most researchers experience that appropriate patients seem to evaporate just as the study is about to start. Lasagna's law predicts that the recruitment rate will fall by at least 50% at just the time your study starts. In general the best way to deal with this is to allow for such predictions in your research planning so that, for example, if your realistic prediction is that you can collect 50 subjects over one year, arrange your study so that your estimated prediction rate can be doubled either by lengthening your recruitment time or by widening your recruitment area.

Some researchers advertise for patients or subjects, and there is nothing wrong with this approach providing you are clear that you will get a quite different subject population from patients recruited via general practitioners or hospital referrals. Much American research is done on this basis and it is often not made clear when projects are written up for publication how patients are recruited. This makes the interpretation of many such studies quite difficult, particularly in the area of depressive, anxiety, and eating disorders. In many studies, subjects are college students who have been advertised for on campus, who bear little similarity to a typical subject referred by a general practitioner in the National Health Service.

One useful way of getting subjects is to offer a service: if for example you are looking for patients with chronic pain, to offer some sort of assessment service or even a treatment programme is one way of ensuring a deluge of referrals.

Replication studies

While it is usually desirable to try to carry out a piece of original research, especially for your first research project, replication studies are very important: it is only when a finding has been replicated in a number of different centres by different investigators that its significance can be properly assessed. There are a number of reasons for this. Firstly, most investigators are not neutral and unbiased, and they embark on research projects because they have a particular idea which they think is correct. In other words, most investigators find what they hope or what they expect to find. It is always worth taking slightly more notice of those studies where a researcher appears to be genuinely surprised by the result obtained or where the results contradict his/her own favoured hypothesis.

Secondly, there is a marked publication bias. Positive studies tend to be reported and published much more frequently than negative ones. It is quite possible for a similar design of study to be carried out in a number of different centres, for the negative results never to see the light of day, and for the one positive result which was atypical to be published. This is not usually deliberate suppression of contradictory data; it is just the understandable desire that researchers and journals have to publish positive findings.

Finally, in any study involving human subjects, one can never be quite sure how representative the subject population is and repeating the study on a different subject population perhaps in a different part of the country or a different environment is always desirable.

The advantage for the trainee of replication studies is that one has a methodology to follow. It is usually possible to contact the original researcher and indicate your desire to repeat the study in a different setting, and most researchers are delighted to collaborate with such endeavours. Do not therefore be ashamed of doing replication studies – they do not constitute second-class research. They are a vitally important part of scientific method.

Coping with failure and how to prevent it

Very few research projects go as planned and a considerable number are never completed. If you do get as far as collecting results, make every effort to write up for publication (see Chapter 12). Do not be too disheartened if you get a negative result. As mentioned earlier, negative results are scientifically just as important as positive ones. It has been suggested, half seriously, that there should be special journals that publish only such negative results and also a journal that publishes the descriptions of research that is abandoned or comes to grief. If it really is impossible for your research project to proceed, then seriously consider writing a paper on a research project that went wrong. There are a few of these in the literature and they provide fascinating reading. Hopefully the chapters that follow will help you design a viable research project and encourage you to carry it through.

There are many reasons that can cause research projects to fail which are outside your control, but to minimise the chance of failure you should at least obey the following rules. Firstly, have a clearly thought-out research design which you have put down on paper and discussed critically with others. Secondly, if at all possible try to arrange to have a supervisor. Thirdly, design your study to collect as much information as you can at the start and as little as possible later. In other words if you are following up patients, try to collect as many details when you first see the patient and keep the amount of data you collect at follow-up interviews to a minimum. Thirdly, try to write your project up as you go along even if it is only in note or diary form as suggested earlier. Fourthly, try to have some sort of fall-back project instead of your main project so that if it goes wrong because of a low response rate, lack of patient recruitment, or for any other reason, then at least you will have a descriptive study or a literature review you can salvage from it.

Having said all this, the two commonest points at which projects fail are firstly that they never get started – the idea is good, the protocol is written but the research never begins – and secondly that all the data are collected, the majority of the work has been done, but then the project results are never analysed and written up. Clearly this is an awful waste of your time and effort but it also has considerable ethical implications. If we carry out research, especially on patients, and we put them to discomfort or at risk, then we have an obligation to see the project through so that the information collected can be shared by others and have a chance of benefiting the patients who originally took part, or of benefiting similar patients in the future.

2 Methodology of clinical trials in psychiatry

TONY JOHNSON

Since its inception in the 1940s, the randomised clinical trial has become the principal method of comparing the efficacy of all forms of medical treatment and care of hospital in-patients, out-patients and in the community. One of its founders, Bradford Hill, described the clinical trial as:

> "a carefully, and ethically, designed experiment with the aim of answering some precisely framed question. In its most rigorous form it demands equivalent groups of patients concurrently treated in different ways. These groups are constructed by the random allocation of patients to one or other treatment. In some instances patients may form their own controls, different treatments being applied to them in random order and the effect compared. In principle the method is applicable with any disease and any treatment." (Hill, 1955)

The distinction between this form of assessment and epidemiological studies is the objective and efficient prospective comparison of concurrent randomly allocated treatments.

Many clinical trials are conducted each year within all specialties of medicine, and these exhibit a range of designs from very simple to highly complex, from tiny to enormous, and from short term to long term, with methods of analysis that vary from the crude to the sophisticated. The past 40 years have seen many developments as researchers have tackled the problems of design of clinical trials, conduct and analysis in attempts to tailor them to the study of specific diseases; methods of assessment, and patient management. Today, there are several comprehensive and readable texts devoted to the methodology of clinical trials, illustrated by examples drawn from the medical literature (see 'Further reading'). There are good reasons for having a text specific to each subspecialty of medicine, so that the problems of actually carrying out clinical trials can be exhibited and discussed as close as possible to their clinical context. Unfortunately, this has happened only rarely (Buyse *et al*, 1984) and so far no detailed text exists within the framework of psychiatry.

The burgeoning methodology of clinical trials has led to some standardisation of terminology to provide a broad classification of the types of trial, the information collected and the way in which it is handled in the analysis. The purpose of this chapter is to present some of the basic terminology and methodology of clinical trials as simply as possible, with illustrations drawn from general psychiatry. In one chapter it is not possible to enter into highly specific details; for these, as well as the arguments for and against various practices and procedures, the reader should consult the list of further reading at the end of this chapter.

The protocol

We begin with the protocol, the construction of which is the first major milestone that must be reached and passed if any clinical trial is organised and carried out successfully. The protocol is not a four- or five-page series of jottings, sketching the purpose of the trial and where it will be conducted, but a complete manual that provides a full specification of the clinical trial, from a statement of its objectives to the writing of the final report. It embraces every aspect of the management and assessment of patients, including copies of forms and rating instruments, together with instructions for their completion and scoring, a summary of the data collected and the methods of computerisation and analysis. Some of the key features of the protocol are listed below.

Title (and abbreviated title)
Objectives: primary aim, secondary aim
Background and rationale
Medical co-ordinator (name, address, telephone number) –
    responsibilities
Statistical co-ordinator (name, address, telephone number) –
    responsibilities
Local co-ordinators' responsibilities
Other specialists – responsibilities
Steering committee – membership and responsibilities
Period of recruitment (starting and finishing dates) and follow-up
Baseline information (demographic, psychiatric history, current illness/
    condition, assessments)
Inclusion and exclusion criteria
Consent
Patient registration
Trial design (stratification, masking, sample size, safety clause)
Randomisation
Administration of treatments
Safety monitoring

Methods of patient follow-up
Assessments and frequency
Discharge from trial on completion
Deviations from protocol
Deaths – post-mortem reports and certificates
Data handling – computerisation and summarisation
Data analysis – statistical power
Progress reports
Publication – authorship
Appendices
   (a) submission to ethics committees
   (b) hand-out for patients and relatives
   (c) patient consent forms
   (d) standardised assessments – instructions for completion and scoring
   (e) trial forms
   (f) flow chart for patients
   (g) flow chart for forms
   (h) participating centres and local co-ordinators

The protocol for a specific clinical trial will not necessarily incorporate all these items, and the order of presentation may be changed. Some investigators use both a protocol and an operators' manual (see Meinert, 1986).

Of these features a few will be singled out for discussion in this chapter. However, the second merits special attention, for many clinical trials in psychiatry are overambitious and attempt to resolve too many, often diverse issues simultaneously. The inevitable result is that inadequate information is obtained about many of them, and investigators are forced to perform rescue operations on selected and perhaps biased data. The primary objective of a clinical trial is the estimation of the difference(s) between the randomised treatments on some chosen measure of efficacy, and this should never be lost sight of. The temptation to investigate secondary objectives on an 'available' sample of patients must be curtailed. The searches for prognostic factors, the identification of the characteristics of 'responders' and 'non-responders', the breakdown of drugs into metabolites and other biochemistry, the development of rating scales and assessments of associations between them, relationships with computerised tomography scans, and so on, are better left to other studies and perhaps more efficient techniques of investigation. Remember Bradford Hill's "precisely framed question" and attempt to answer it (and little else) as simply as possible.

Clinical trials conducted at just one hospital, one clinic or in one practice, by a single investigator are termed single-centre trials; by contrast multicentre trials recruit patients from two, or usually more, settings. However, the distinction between the two is not always clear and, for example, may be confused when patients at just one hospital are entered by independent physicians or clinics. The protocol must list the principal investigator as well as the collaborating centres together with the names of the co-ordinating physicians. The number of hospitals/clinics should be justified by sensible estimates of the rates of patient recruitment and the choice of sample size, the latter determined objectively, for example by a power calculation.

The statistical co-ordinator

All clinical trials should be carried out in conjunction with a statistical co-ordinator, whose functions include those listed below.

> Selection of clinical trial design
> Selection of response variables
> Determination of sample size
> Estimates of recruitment rates and numbers of participating centres
> Design of clinical trial forms
> Design and analysis of pilot studies
> Determination of method of randomisation
> Implementation of selected randomisation scheme
> Checking and computerisation of clinical trial data
> Validation of clinical trial data
> Analysis of data
> Summarisation of data and analysis

These details must appear in the protocol. Ideally it should be possible for an independent team of investigators to take over the organisation and running of a clinical trial to the extent of completing and publishing it as planned, after reading and studying the protocol alone.

The pilot study

Since the conduct of any clinical trial is a very complicated exercise in the management of patients, it is sensible to ensure that important logistic elements in the protocol have been tested adequately before the trial commences. Such testing is often carried out within a pilot study, especially to check the design of forms, the recruitment of patients, indistinguishability of treatments in a blind design, and handling of the data. However, the objectives of a pilot study should not be too much; for example, they are not suitable for the design of rating instruments, which constitutes a research project in itself!

Pilot studies would have identified problems encountered by Blackwell & Shepherd (1967), who recruited only eight patients out of 518 admitted to the two participating centres; Cook *et al* (1988) encountered problems of organisation, management, conception of treatment and finance. Both reports are highly instructive and worthy of detailed study.

Recruitment rates

The principal difficulty encountered in the design of most trials is the accurate

TABLE 2.1
Examples of entry criteria from some recent clinical trials

Inclusion criteria	Exclusion criteria
Depression in women in general practice (Corney, 1987)	
Women aged 18–45 years	Major physical ill health
Referred by one of six designated general practitioners	Already under treatment by social worker
	Preferred treatment
Acute depression in previous 3 months or chronic depression intensified in previous 3 months	
Score of 2 or more on Clinical Interview Schedule	
Consent to randomisation and follow-up	
Unipolar depression in in-patients and out-patients (Glen *et al*, 1984)	
Aged 25–65	History of mania
Attending/referred to 9 designated centres	Contra-indication to randomised treatment
Diagnosis of primary depressive illness (defined) lasting at least 1 month	
Consent to randomisation	
Confusion in the elderly (Baines *et al*, 1987)	
Resident at a specific local authority home for the elderly	Severe communication problem
Confused	Preferred treatment
Moderate/severe impairment of cognitive function (Clifton Assessment Procedures for the Elderly)	
Consent to randomisation	
Out-patients with schizophrenia (Johnson *et al*, 1987)	
Consecutive out-patients at specific centre diagnosed with schizophrenia and satisfying Feighner criteria	Organic brain disease
	Physical illness
	Alcohol or substance abuse
Total score less than 4 on the Brief Psychiatric Rating Scale	Below normal IQ
	Additional mental illness
Maintained on low doses of flupenthixol decanoate for previous year and stable dose not exceeding 40 mg per 2 weeks over past 6 months	Preferred treatment
Consent to randomisation	
Melancholia and dysthymic disorder in out-patients (Vallejo *et al*, 1987)	
Unmedicated psychiatric out-patients attending specific clinics	Severe physical disorder
	On-going medical treatment
Aged 18–63	Pregnancy
Major depressive episode with melancholia or dysthymic disorder (DSM–III)	Psychopathic/sociopathic disorder
	Briquet's syndrome
	Alcohol/drug abuse
Hamilton Rating Scale for Depression score >16	Psychotic illness
Consent to randomisation	Bipolar, obsessive–compulsive, somatiform, panic, eating, or phobic disorder (DSM–III)

continued

TABLE 2.1 *continued*

Persistent generalised anxiety (Butler *et al*, 1987)

Referrals from specific general practitioners or psychiatric out-patient clinics	Satisfies Research Diagnostic Criteria for phobic, obsessive–compulsive or major depressive disorder
Generalised anxiety disorder (GAD) or panic disorder with primary GAD as defined by Research Diagnostic Criteria	Chronic anxiety with no period of 1 month in last 2 years of symptoms
Score of 7 or more on Leeds Anxiety Scale	Preferred treatment
Current episode of anxiety lasted at least 6 months	
Consent to randomisation	

Adapted from the papers quoted; not all of them give 'consent to randomisation' among the inclusion criteria, or 'preferred treatment' among the exclusion criteria.

estimation of recruitment rates, even with the benefits of pilot studies. Indeed it is often said ruefully by clinical researchers that if you wish to reduce the impact of a disorder you need only carry out a clinical trial of its treatment; all the suitable patients will then disappear! In view of this it is sensible to incorporate a safety clause within the protocol itself; this will result in the abandonment of the trial if the recruitment of patients over an initial specified period is below a designated target.

Sample

The patients entered in a clinical trial form a sample selected from some much larger population. The characteristics of both the population and the sample, as well as the method of selection, must be defined precisely so that the results from the clinical trial can be used in making decisions about the care of future patients. Strictly speaking, the sample should be selected *randomly* from a defined population but this is rarely possible in clinical trials, for ethical reasons. Consequently it is impossible to establish the specific nature of the population represented by the chosen sample, and necessary to make some broad, although not necessarily unreasonable, assumptions in generalising the results of the clinical trial. Standardised instruments, such as the Brief Psychiatric Rating Scale, and Hamilton Rating Scales for Depression and Anxiety, as well as diagnostic instruments such as DSM–III and the Present State Examination (see Chapter 9), are useful in characterising patients entered in a clinical trial and may serve in the selection of a reasonably homogeneous sample of patients. The inverse process of deciding whether the results from a trial can guide treatment of a particular patient is a less structured process requiring clinical intuition and judgement.

Entry criteria

The sample and population are specified in terms of inclusion and exclusion criteria, known collectively as entry criteria, which determine the patients who should be considered for entry to the trial as well as those who are actually entered. There is no specific rule for choosing whether a criterion is inclusive (for example selecting patients in the age range 20–65 years) or exclusive (leaving out patients less than 20 or older than 65). In practice it is convenient to establish the broad category of patients intended to be treated by the inclusion criteria and to use the exclusion criteria to establish contra-indications; examples appear in Table 2.1. The exclusion criteria must embrace patients for whom the caring psychiatrist has a preferred treatment as well as patients who do not consent to randomisation. Patients in either of these two categories inevitably introduce some nebulosity into the entry criteria since it is extremely difficult to quantify the reasons for a preferred treatment and virtually impossible to establish the personal reasons for rejecting randomisation. Perhaps the best that can be achieved is to report the numbers of such patients. The other inclusion and exclusion criteria should be specified precisely using recognised definitions and established instruments.

Data

The information about patients considered for entry into a clinical trial may be divided into several categories: first, the basic demographic data, which describe the broad characteristics of the sample, for example sex, age, social class and residence; second, the medical history, which summarises relevant aspects of previous diseases and treatments; third, clinical details of the illness or condition that led to consideration for entry to the trial; fourth, monitoring information about the treatment of patients in a trial; and finally, information on the progress of the disease or condition, which will form the basis for the comparison of treatments.

Variables

To the statistician any item of information or characteristic that may vary from one patient to another, or which may vary within one patient from one time to another, is termed a variable. Variables can be subdivided into different types, each of which requires specific methods of summarisation and analysis. The principal types are:

(a) continuous (e.g. age), which can take any value within a limited range
(b) binary (dichotomous), such as sex (male, female) and patient status (in-patient/out-patient), which can take only one of two values
(c) categorical (polychotomous), such as hospital of treatment or diagnostic group
(d) ordinal such as age group, or response to treatment (worse, none, improved), where there is a natural ordering of the categories.

Variables can sometimes be transferred from one category to another by recoding, thus enabling alternative methods of summarisation and statistical modelling. For example, rating scales such as the Hamilton Rating Scale for Depression can be analysed as continuous variables using the actual (or perhaps transformed) score, as an ordinal variable by recoding into groups (less than 10, 11–19, 20–29, or at least 30), or as a binary variable by defining a cut-off point (less than 15, at least 15).

As well as subdividing variables by types in the statistical sense above, it is convenient in clinical trials to subdivide them according to their status in the analysis. Data about patients collected before randomisation (which is usually taken as the time of entry to a clinical trial) as well as the allocated treatment itself are called baseline variables; other collective nouns, such as concomitant and independent variables, covariates and covariables, are sometimes used, although some of these have specialised interpretations in the context of statistical analysis. Data collected to assess compliance with treatment such as tablet counts and blood or serum concentrations are called, quite naturally, monitoring variables, while the measures used to assess the effects of treatment, including side-effects, are referred to as response or outcome variables; monitoring and response variables collectively may be called follow-up variables.

Blinding

In many clinical trials of treatment, particularly for psychiatric patients, in whom there is some subjectivity in both disease definition and quantification of response, it is necessary to make the assessment of response as objective as possible. In practice this is helped by masking or blinding the assessor to the identity of the allocated treatment. Trials in which one assessor (patient or clinician) is masked are called single blind; when both are masked they are double blind. When the results from laboratory assays are reported back to the managing physicians in standardised (or coded) units, thus not revealing the identity of the treatment, the trial may be termed triple blind. However, triple blindness may also be used to refer to other aspects of masking, for example not revealing the identity of treatment to the data analysts. Clinical trials where there is no attempt to disguise the nature or form of treatment either to the patient or to the managing physicians are termed open studies.

Forms and computers

Information about patients entered into clinical trials is recorded on specially designed forms and ultimately transferred to a computer for storage and analysis (Ch. 13). Each step of the process of eliciting, recording and transferring information may introduce inaccuracies (errors and miscodings) into the data actually analysed, and no amount of checking and rechecking will eliminate all of them. The best practice is to simplify each step.

Forms should be designed primarily to aid patient assessment and accurate recording, and secondarily to enable easy transfer of information to a computer; there are a number of principles which should be observed (Wright & Haybittle, 1979; Gore, 1981a; Meinert, 1986). Perhaps the most important are that separate forms should be used for each source of information (one for baseline clinical interview, another for standardised ratings, a third for baseline biochemistry and laboratory assays, and yet others for follow-up information); they should have a unified (same print style) and above all simple format (not too many items per page), with data entry towards one side, usually the right. The layout of forms for clinical interview should follow the natural order of information retrieval and patient assessment, and standard rating instruments borrowed from external sources should be recast in the style and format of other study forms. Transfer of data to computer (as well as summarisation and analysis) is aided by structuring the form to provide a standardised response to each question and the liberal use of boxes either for the recording of numerical information or to be ticked; the boxes should not be too small (at least 8 mm square) and aligned both horizontally and vertically.

It should be possible to transfer information directly from the forms to a computer. This can be achieved with a computer database (for example dBase 3 Plus, DataEase and SPSSPC+) which may provide an identical image of the form itself, or by direct entry to a standard computer file. Before using any database on a personal or microcomputer, make sure that the data can be output in a standard (ASCII) file, for the latter can be read by a larger (mainframe) computer, which may be required during analysis. Computer files should be structured so that they provide a usable manual record; this is achieved by the insertion of a blank field between blocks of data (about one blank for every 10–15 characters) rather than entering data across every column of the record.

It is not always appreciated that it is unnecessary to convert all information to numerical digits (0–9) in computer records; alphanumeric characters (letters as well as numbers) can be used, are visually informative and help limit coding errors, for example using 'SCH' for schizophrenia, 'ANX' for anxiety, and so on, instead of recoding to numbers such as 01, 02, etc. This can be performed by the computer. When feasible, data should be stored in a basic form (date of birth, date of previous admission) rather than a derived form (age, period from last admission) which is subject to the inaccuracies of mental arithmetic; leave the calculations to the computer! Unstructured data, especially unsolicited comments and anecdotal information, should not be entered into a computer file; if desired its presence on forms can be flagged by an indicator in the computer record. (A blank field for no comment and 1 to denote some comment.) Personal data (name and/or address) that could lead to easy identification of patients from a display unit or printed output should not be entered into the computer; use an identity number in the computer record and keep a master list of names and identity numbers in a secure place.

No one should be daunted by the prospect of using a terminal, even if it is connected to a large computer. The ubiquity of personal computers has made their operation familiar to most. However, data summarisation and analysis pose many problems. Packages such as SPSS, BMDP and SAS (see Appendix) enable most users to produce prestigious volumes of output, much of which will be but vaguely comprehensible to the uninitiated. These three packages (with the addition of GLIM and GENSTAT) are sufficient for the analysis of almost all clinical trial data but preferably in consultation with a statistician.

One of the worst spin-offs from the ready availability of large computers (and comparatively cheap computation) is the belief that these machines can fairly easily summarise and analyse almost unlimited volumes of data, much of it of quite dubious quality. Many clinical trials attempt to collect far too much information, and researchers discover only at the end that their data do not serve the purposes of the study or that the structure of the data is too complex to provide a convincing analysis. Most would appreciate intuitively that it is difficult to place much reliance on statements about the inter-relationships between 100 different items of information collected from just ten individuals, yet in many clinical trials the ratio of variables to patients may be on this scale. It is sometimes advised that the ratio of subjects to variables should exceed five, ten, or the actual number of variables. While the origin of such rules is obscure, they provide some guidance to sensible analysis. And remember that the total score from a rating scale will count as one variable, while the analysis of each component item (item analysis) counts as many variables as items.

Stratification

Quite often it is known before the start of a clinical trial that some of the baseline variables influence response to treatment. For example neurotic and endogenous subtypes of depression affect response to antidepressants, while the period of onset of schizophrenia is related to recurrence of psychotic symptoms. Such variables are called prognostic variables or prognostic factors. In any clinical trial it would be unfortunate if a majority of patients with good prognosis were concentrated in one treatment group. Simple comparisons of response between the treatment groups would then be biased by the imbalance of the prognostic factor. One of the purposes of randomisation is to guard against such imbalance, and the bias it produces. Since even with randomisation it is possible that there will be some imbalance, investigators often prefer to ensure that the bias from known prognostic factors is minimised by pre-stratification, that is, stratification before randomisation. Essentially patients are split into groups ('strata') defined by the levels (or some combination of levels) of an important prognostic (stratifying) variable; assignment to treatment is then carried out randomly within each stratum. More than one stratifying variable can be chosen although there is no point in selecting more than three or four. In multicentre trials it is standard practice to pre-stratify patients by centre, partly because it is likely that patients at one will have a different prognosis from those at another, but partly to avoid the awkwardness and suspicion that results from treatment imbalances within centres.

As an alternative to pre-stratification, the comparison of treatments can always be adjusted in the analysis for any variable considered of prognostic importance (given sufficient patients in the trial) provided it has been recorded as a baseline variable; this technique is known as post-stratification. In view of this facility some statisticians recommend that large clinical trials should be performed by abandoning pre-stratification altogether. Frequently the combination of pre- and post-stratification is useful in the same trial.

Randomisation

It has been acknowledged for many years that the only satisfactory method of assigning treatments in a clinical trial is by randomisation. Today no other method is acceptable, for reasons that are well presented in many textbooks. Here we are concerned not with reasons for randomisation but with just two of the many ways by which the process may be carried out, namely the sealed-envelope technique, and the method of minimisation. Whichever method is chosen, it should be set up in consultation with a statistical co-ordinator who cannot only maintain it but also check that the system is not abused. Sealed envelopes are prepared by a statistician and may be used to allocate treatment from a central organisation (by the medical investigator or, preferably, the statistical co-ordinator) or at individual centres by the co-ordinating physicians; the method of minimisation requires a central organisation. When sealed envelopes are distributed to centres it is difficult to maintain a detailed check of whether patients have been entered in the trial or excluded, unless randomisation can be carried out by a department such as the pharmacy, which is independent of the clinical trial. For this reason and others, centralisation of the logging of patient entry and randomisation is preferred; the entire process can be accomplished efficiently by telephone, and hence it is known as telephone registration or telephone randomisation.

On entry to a clinical trial patients are allotted a trial number, which serves as a unique identifier on all records (both written forms and letters, and computer files). Trial numbers should have a simple format with a constant number of characters not exceeding four. The first character may be a letter used to identify the centre in a multicentre trial. For example one letter combined with two digits allows 23 centres each entering up to 99 patients.

(Note that the letters I, O and Z are excluded to avoid confusion with the numbers 1, 0 and 2.) The trial numbers are then recorded to the same fixed length, e.g. B01 (*not* B1) D12.

The sealed-envelope technique

This technique (Gore, 1981) is practicable in clinical trials with a small number of stratifying factors and a small number of strata. It is usually convenient to number the individual strata sequentially and then prepare a separate batch of envelopes for each. The envelopes are given a serial number within each stratum and ordered sequentially, starting from 1. It is usual to label the envelope with the title of the trial (perhaps abbreviated), the number of the stratum and an abbreviated description of the stratum characteristics, as well as the serial number. Each envelope contains a card labelled with the same information as the corresponding envelope together with the identity of the treatment allocated. In addition, the cards may have space to enter the patient's name and trial number as well as the date of randomisation; they may be colour coded and used as an index of patients entered in the trial. Envelopes are kept and opened in strictly increasing order of the serial numbers in each stratum; only one envelope is used per patient and is opened only *after* the decision to randomise treatment has been made. The envelopes are usually destroyed after opening. The treatments designated on the cards are determined using random permuted blocks, to ensure that the numbers of patients allocated to each treatment are balanced within each stratum at predetermined, but not necessarily constant, intervals.

It will be appreciated that the preparation of cards and envelopes can result in a considerable amount of work. For this reason, and others, the method of minimisation (White & Freedman, 1978; Gore, 1981*b*) may be preferred. However, the workload in preparing batches of cards may be reduced by using the cheque-book principle. Initially a small batch of cards is prepared for each stratum. About three-quarters of the way through each batch there appears a contrasting envelope containing a letter of request for further cards; after the preceding envelope in the batch has been opened and used to allocate treatment, this letter is sent to the statistical co-ordinator, who responds promptly with a further batch of envelopes for that stratum (including another request for further cards). The sizes of the second and subsequent batches can be adjusted according to the recruitment rate in the stratum.

The method of randomisation is illustrated in Fig. 2.1 for an open clinical trial of amitriptyline compared with mianserin in patients with manic–depressive psychosis; patients are stratified by centre (hospitals, A, B and C), sex, and the number of previous episodes of affective disorder (less than three/three or more), giving three stratifying factors with three, two and two levels respectively. The total number of strata is then 12 ($3 \times 2 \times 2$). Thus 12 separate series of randomisation envelopes are prepared. If randomisation is centralised, the 12 series will be kept together at one

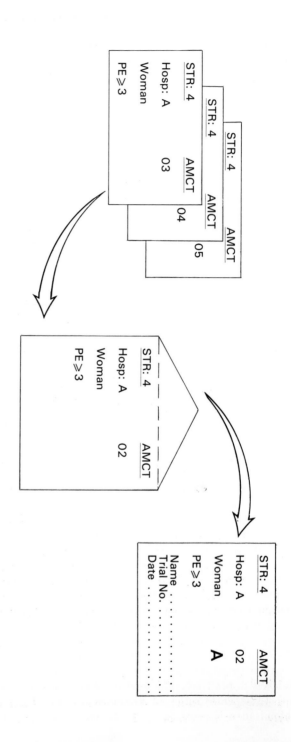

Fig. 2.1 Randomisation by the sealed-envelope technique. The second patient in stratum (STR) 4, a woman with at least three previous episodes (PE) of affective disorder under treatment at hospital (Hosp) A is allocated A(mitriptyline). Abbreviated clinical trial title: AMCT

TABLE 2.2

Treatment allocations for the first 20 patients entered in a hypothetical clinical trial comparing the efficacy of amitriptyline and mianserin in manic–depressive psychosis

Patient	Hospital	Sex	No. of previous affective episodes	Trial no.	Allocated treatment
1	A	F	1	A01	Mianserin
2	B	F	1	B01	Amitriptyline
3	A	F	2	A02	Amitriptyline
4	C	M	4	C01	Amitriptyline
5	C	F	2	C02	Mianserin
6	A	M	2	A03	Mianserin
7	A	F	2	A04	Amitriptyline
8	B	M	1	B02	Mianserin
9	A	F	2	A05	Amitriptyline
10	A	F	3	A06	Mianserin
11	C	F	6	C03	Mianserin
12	A	M	3	A07	Amitriptyline
13	C	F	2	C04	Amitriptyline
14	B	F	2	B03	Mianserin
15	B	F	4	B04	Amitriptyline
16	A	M	2	A08	Mianserin
17	A	F	1	A09	Amitriptyline
18	C	F	3	C05	Mianserin
19	A	M	2	A10	Mianserin
20	A	M	2	A11	Amitriptyline
21	A	F	3	?	?

The 21st patient is the 12th to enter the trial from hospital A, the second patient with the combination of characteristics – hospital A, female sex and at least three affective episodes. Her trial number is A12. The allocation of treatment is discussed under 'Randomisation'.

location, whereas with local randomisation four separate series of envelopes will be distributed to each of the three centres. We assume that 20 patients have been entered in the trial with the characteristics, trial numbers and allocated treatments shown in Table 2.2. The next patient to enter (number 21) is a woman with three previous episodes of affective disorder under treatment at hospital A; being the 12th patient to enter from this centre she receives trial number A12. Since she is the second female patient at hospital A with at least three affective episodes (a combination which we will assume characterises stratum 4), her treatment is allocated by opening envelope number 2 of the series for this stratum. Fig. 2.1 shows that this patient is prescribed A(mitriptyline). Special care is required when using this method in double-blind trials to ensure that treatment is identified uniquely for each patient, so that there is no possibility of disclosure of the treatment given to a whole group of patients if the code is broken for one.

The method of minimisation

An alternative technique to sealed envelopes and one that is generally preferred is the method of minimisation, which aims to minimise some

Hospital A			
A	M	A	M
A02	A01		
A04	A03		
A05	A06		
A07	A08		
A09	A10		
A11			

Imbalance with allocation to:

A(mitriptyline)   M(ianserin)

$7 - 5 = 2$ $6 - 6 = 0$

Women			
A	M	A	M
B01	A01		
A02	C02		
A04	A06		
A05	C03		
C04	B03		
B04	C05		
A09			

$8 - 6 = 2$ $7 - 7 = 0$

Previous episodes $\geqslant 3$			
A	M	A	M
C01	A06		
A07	C03		
B04	C05		

$4 - 3 = 1$ $4 - 3 = 1$

Overall imbalance:
                    5   1

Fig. 2.2   *Randomisation by the method of minimisation. Patient 21 (see Table 2.3) is allocated mianserin since the overall imbalance of 1 is smaller than with amitriptyline*

measure of imbalance between the numbers of patients assigned to the different treatments over each of the stratifying factors. The method requires some centralisation of the randomisation procedure and may be implemented in several different ways; we present just one of these. A separate card is prepared for each stratum and used to indicate the numbers of patients within that stratum assigned to each treatment (usually by entering the trial number). When a patient is entered into the trial the cards for the corresponding strata are selected, the measure of imbalance is calculated with the new patient assigned to each treatment in turn, and the treatment which leads to the least imbalance is allocated. The whole process should take less than one minute.

The method is illustrated for the example above in Fig. 2.2, where the patient to be entered in the trial is again number 21, a woman with three previous episodes of affective disorder under treatment at hospital A. We assume that our measure of imbalance is just the absolute difference between the total numbers of patients assigned to each treatment summed over the appropriate strata. The three cards for 'hospital A', 'women' and 'at least three affective episodes' are selected. Assignment of patient A12 to amitriptyline gives imbalances of $7 - 5 = 2$, $8 - 6 = 2$ and $4 - 3 = 1$ on these three cards and a total imbalance of $2 + 2 + 1 = 5$; assignment to mianserin leads to a total imbalance of $(6 - 6) + (7 - 7) + (4 - 3) = 0 + 0 + 1$. The smaller imbalance is achieved if the patient is assigned mianserin. If the total imbalance had been equal for the two treatments, the allocation could be made using a table of random assignments.

There are many variants of this method, some of them superior to the one described above. It is possible to use alternative measures of imbalance, and to apply different weights to the imbalance for each stratifying factor. In addition, treatment assignment may incorporate biased randomisation even when there is overall imbalance so that the procedure is not entirely predictable.

Design of trials

There are only a few basic designs used in clinical trials, although there are many variations upon them. At one extreme lie the *fixed sample size* trials, in which the number of patients recruited is decided at the design stage, and at the other lie the *fully sequential* trials, which proceed until some predetermined termination (or stopping) criterion or rule is fulfilled. With fixed sample size trials, in principle, there should be just one single analysis at the predefined endpoint of the study, whereas in sequential trials analysis is repeated as the results of patient assessment become available. In practice, with fixed sample size trials, especially those including prolonged follow-up or requiring patient recruitment to extend over more than one year, there are often repeat ('interim') analyses of response to treatment, which have not been anticipated at the design stage and which make no allowance for multiple 'looks' at the data (multiple comparisons). Such practices are undesirable since they inflate the false positive (or type I error) rate (see 'Power and confidence', below). To resolve this problem a new class of 'group sequential designs' (Pocock, 1978) was introduced, in which analyses are repeated at regular intervals throughout the trial; the maximum number of analyses is determined at the design stage. Here we restrict attention to just two types of fixed sample size trial, namely parallel group and cross-over designs. However, first we introduce some terminology which is common to all trial designs.

Patients

All patients considered for entry to a clinical trial are assessed at a screening examination, which may be extended over a baseline period of observation and evaluation, before randomisation. Patients who do not satisfy the entry criteria for the trial are obviously ineligible, and are not usually pursued further; patients who satisfy all the entry criteria except those concerned with agreement to randomisation, and consequently are eligible to participate in the trial, may be subdivided into two groups: those patients who agree to participate (that is give informed consent), who become trial entrants; and the eligible patients who do not consent to take part, sometimes referred to as eligible non-randomised patients. Although these latter patients

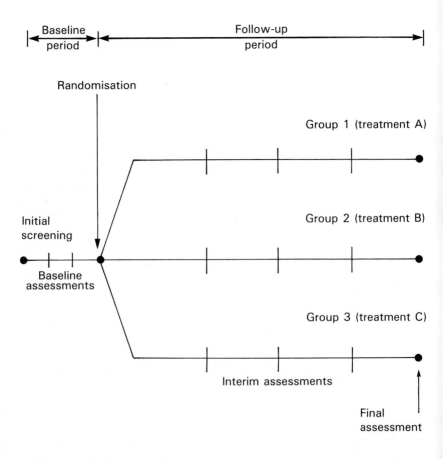

Fig. 2.3   Parallel group clinical trials. The standard fixed size three-treatment parallel group design. Patients are screened, assessed over a baseline period, and randomised to one of three treatment groups. The follow-up period may either be of set duration as illustrated here or, especially in clinical trials with extended follow-up, may vary from patient to patient

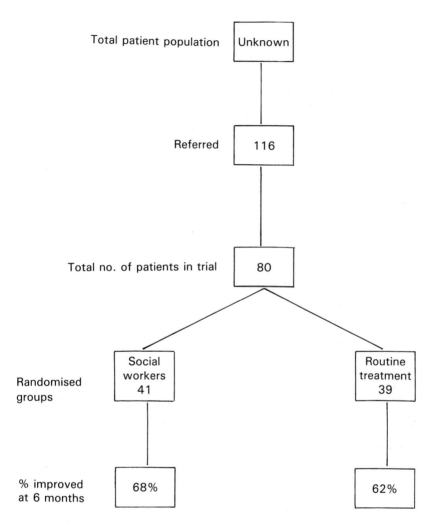

Total patient population | Unknown

Referred | 116

Total no. of patients in trial | 80

Social workers 41   Routine treatment 39

Randomised groups

% improved at 6 months | 68% | 62%

Fig. 2.4   A randomised, parallel group trial of social worker intervention in depressed women patients in general practice. Patients were assessed at six months (and again at one year) (for full details see Corney (1987))

play no further part in the clinical trial itself and certainly cannot contribute to the assessment of efficacy, they are important in defining the population of patients to whom the results of the study may be applied. Keeping a log of these patients as well as details of the baseline variables thus enables the identification of systematic differences between trial entrants and eligible non-randomised patients.

Parallel group trials

In parallel group trials patients are allocated at random to one of two, or perhaps more, treatment groups and should be followed up and assessed in the manner dictated by the trial design. Usually this implies that patients will be followed up for a set period, or until a specific calendar day; long-term trials may incorporate a mixture of the two. The follow-up evaluations include interim assessments after specified periods and final assessments, when patients are formally discharged from the clinical trial; sometimes there are no interim assessments. The information collected at interim assessments is usually standardised but frequently varies from one assessment to another; for example, in studies of antidepressant drugs, ratings of the severity of depression may be obtained weekly, whereas biochemistry may be performed only every two weeks. One basic format is shown in Fig. 2.3. The main analysis of such trials compares summary measures of response in the different treatment groups.

An example is provided by Corney (1987), who investigated the effectiveness of social work intervention in depressed patients in general practice; 80 women who agreed to take part in the clinical trial were allocated randomly to routine treatment by their general practitioners or referral to attached social workers. The women were assessed on entry to the study using the Clinical Interview Schedule and the Social Maladjustment Schedule, and reassessed after six months and one year. A simplified schematic representation (Hampton, 1981) of the results at six months is presented in Fig. 2.4.

An example of a different type is a clinical trial of continuation therapy in unipolar depressive illness in which 136 patients were randomly allocated to prophylactic treatment with lithium, amitriptyline, or placebo on recovery from a depressive episode, and followed for three years or until relapse (Glen *et al*, 1984) (Fig. 2.5). This study demonstrates both actuarial techniques, which are particularly relevant for the analysis of clinical trials requiring prolonged observation of each patient, and the pragmatic approach of comparing treatment policies by analysis based on the 'intention to treat' (see Peto *et al*, 1975, 1976; and 'Clinical trials in practice', below).

Cross-over trials

In a cross-over trial patients receive more than one treatment, and whereas response in a parallel group study is assessed from differences *between* the patients in different treatment groups, here the response is assessed from treatment differences in the same patients. Since the treatments are given sequentially within a short time span, they cannot be curative and are best chosen for the treatment of conditions associated with an underlying chronic disease. The basic two-period, two-treatment design is shown in Fig. 2.6. Patients are screened and assessed for entry in a similar manner to the parallel

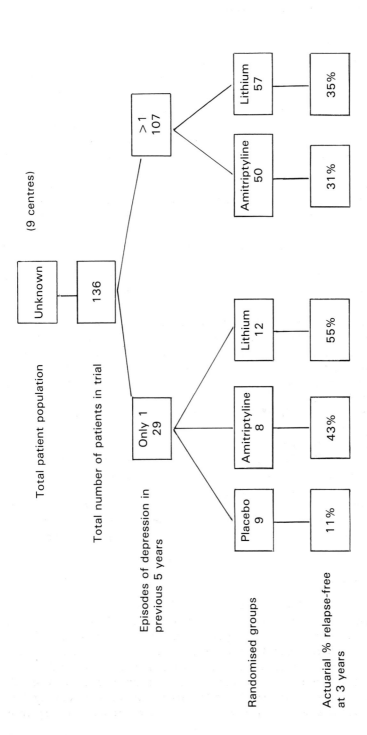

Fig. 2.5   Medical Research Council randomised double-blind parallel group trial of continuation therapy in unipolar depressive illness. A pragmatic trial analysed by 'intention to treat' with patients followed for three years or until relapse (for details see Glen et al, 1984)

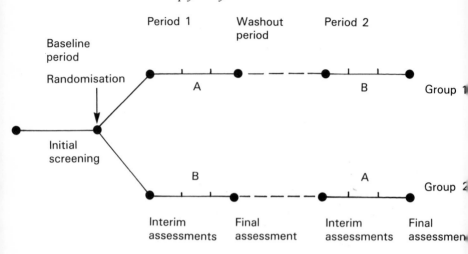

Fig. 2.6   *The standard two-period two-treatment cross-over trial: patients are screened, assessed over a baseline period, and randomised to one of two treatment sequences, either treatment A, washout, and treatment B (group 1), or treatment B, washout, and treatment A (group 2)*

group study, and trial entrants are randomised to group 1, who receive treatment A during period 1 followed by treatment B during period 2, or to group 2, who receive treatment B during period 1 and treatment A during period 2. There is often a 'washout period' between the two treatments, the main purpose of which is to eliminate the effect of treatment given in period 1 before starting treatment in period 2. It may also be used to repeat some baseline observations so that response to treatment can be expressed in terms of changes from a baseline, rather than in absolute values. The treatment periods are of the same duration and have the same pattern of interim followed by final assessments. The duration of the treatment periods need not be disclosed to patients or assessors, who would then be 'blind' to the actual cross-over period. In principle the design may be extended to include more than two treatment periods, more than two treatments, and more than two treatment sequences; such extensions are rare because of the severe logistic problems of actually following up the patients and the difficulties in analysis that result from patient default.

As an illustration, Fig. 2.7 shows the plan of an extended cross-over trial of reality orientation and reminiscence therapy in 15 elderly confused people (Baines *et al*, 1987). The five people in group C constitute a parallel control group. The cross-over is formed from the five people in group A, who received four weeks of reality orientation followed by four weeks without therapy and then four weeks of reminiscence therapy, and the five people in group B, who received a similar programme of therapy but with reminiscence therapy first. Five response measures were used and were

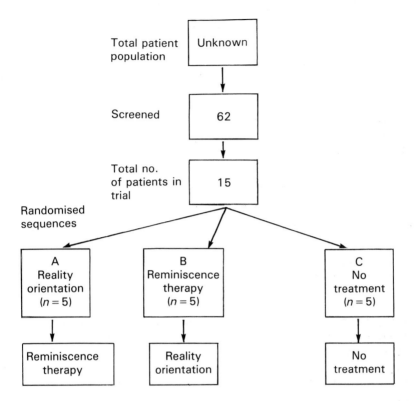

Fig. 2.7 Extended cross-over trial of reality orientation and reminiscence therapy in elderly confused people. The first two sequences form the cross-over; the third sequence is a 'no treatment' control. The treatment periods lasted four weeks and were separated by four weeks. Assessment of six measures of outcome were made at four-weekly intervals from the start of the trial (for full details see Baines et al *(1987)). In conventional cross-over trials, only the two randomised treatment sequences are included. The 'no treatment' controls are an elaboration not necessary for the comparison of the two forms of therapy*

assessed at four-weekly intervals up to 16 weeks. It should have been appreciated at the design stage that the sample size was inadequate.

Choice of design

The selection of a specific design for any clinical trial must be decided in consultation with a medical statistician. This discussion focuses not merely on the choice between a fixed sized or sequential parallel group design, or cross-over trial, but extends to assessment of response, frequency of data collection, sample size, recruitment period and, indeed, any of the other functions listed on page 15. Design must be dictated not merely by the diseases and treatments under evaluation, but also by the exigencies of clinical practice. Nonetheless there are fundamental differences between the three basic designs mentioned above and some guidance about their use may be helpful.

Fully sequential designs (Armitage, 1975) are restricted to the very simple situation where there are just two treatments under comparison by a *single* measure of response or outcome, and where assessment is fairly rapid, at least by comparison with the period of patient entry. They are designed to provide rapid comparative assessment of outcome especially when there are important differences in efficacy between treatments. Apart from requiring the specification of a stopping rule, they have two major disadvantages in that it is difficult both to incorporate information on prognostic factors and to assess efficacy on responses other than that selected at the design stage. Their major advantage over a comparable fixed size, parallel group trial lies in the exposure of fewer patients to an inferior treatment. Sequential trials have been used very rarely in psychiatry (see Joyce & Welldon (1965) for an interesting yet contentious example and Feely *et al* (1982) for a contemporary example comparing clobazam (a benzodiazepine) with placebo in the suppression of seizures associated with menstruation).

In cross-over trials at least two treatments are administered sequentially to each patient and such designs are therefore useless in conditions or diseases such as anxiety and depression, which may be relieved for long and unpredictable periods by treatment. They may be useful in studying relief of side-effects such as Parkinsonism associated with the administration of neuroleptic medication for schizophrenia, or indeed the relief of any acute condition associated with underlying chronic disease. However, they may give rise to ethical problems with the exchange of one treatment for another in patients who benefit from the treatment first administered, and they are sabotaged by patients who default during the first period of treatment (and are not available to receive the second). Because of problems associated with the prolonged observation of patients, cross-over trials should incorporate treatment periods which are reasonably short and rarely exceed six weeks. Their appeal stems from the beguiling assumption that since the differences between treatments are evaluated *within* patients they require far fewer participants than a comparable parallel group study. This may indeed be true but only under quite restrictive assumptions about the absence of differential carry-over effects (Hills & Armitage, 1979; Millar, 1983). The extension of cross-over trials to three or more treatments allows estimation of, and adjustment for, differential carry-over effects from one period of treatment to another, but only at a price of an even more extended trial and the administration of multiple treatments.

By far the most popular of all trial designs is the fixed sample, parallel group study which can be adapted, usually quite easily, to the study of any treatment, however diverse, in any disease. Most issues of all general psychiatric journals which have appeared over the past ten years contain at least one example. The design should be the first choice for any clinical trial in psychiatry and abandoned in favour of a cross-over trial only after careful appraisal. Their main practical disadvantage lies in the requirement for comparatively large numbers of patients, which may result in a recruitment period extended over several years. Such problems can be resolved by proper estimation of recruitment rates at the design stage and collaboration between centres in a multicentre trial.

Clinical trials in practice

No clinical trial is perfect either in design or execution, for no matter how carefully planned and conducted, the actual behaviour of patients as well as the data collected will be somewhat different from those originally envisaged. Just a few of the problems that should be anticipated are shown in Fig. 2.8.

Patients who default during the baseline period before randomisation do not constitute a source of bias in the comparison of treatments, although they do pose a problem for recruitment to the trial if their numbers are substantial. Trial entrants who complete the schedule as detailed in the protocol are sometimes referred to as 'compliers', 'trial compliers' or 'completers', whereas those who do not are 'non-compliers', 'non-completers' or 'trial deviants'. This second group may be subdivided further into those patients who are followed up and assessed as required by the study design, but whose treatment is changed because of side-effects, those patients who simply do not take treatment as scheduled, and patients who do not complete the scheduled assessments, who are referred to as 'losses to follow-up'. Collectively these patients are 'deviations from protocol' or 'deviations from treatment'; the terms 'withdrawals from treatment' or 'withdrawals from protocol' are also used frequently, but should be avoided since they give the misleading impression that such patients are simply taken out of the trial at the time of deviation and are not followed up further. Occasionally patients who do not satisfy the entry criteria are randomised into a clinical trial; this may arise quite simply by mistake (i.e. entered in error) or because it later becomes clear that the patient has a different disease or condition to that specified by the protocol.

It is apparent that the problems described above and illustrated in Fig. 2.8 are just those encountered in the routine management of patients under normal clinical care. The designer of any clinical trial will then be faced with a major quandary in deciding whether to eliminate the non-compliers by intensive patient management or simply to assess the treatments as used in practice. Either approach requires elimination as far as possible of the losses to follow-up for which only death (or perhaps migration) are reasonable excuses.

Explanatory and pragmatic trials

The two extremes are represented by explanatory trials and pragmatic trials. The objective of an explanatory trial is to answer a scientific question about

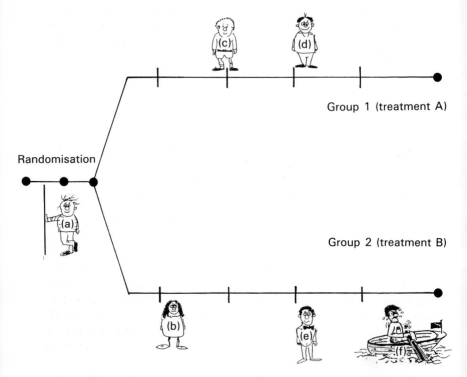

Fig. 2.8   Clinical trials in practice. Some of the problems which arise frequently in practice, illustrated in the context of a two-treatment parallel group design:

(a) defaults during baseline period (not randomised)
(b) discovered subsequently to have another disease/condition (entered in error)
(c) randomised to group 1 (treatment A) but given treatment B
(d) side-effects of treatment, dose reduced
(e) defaults interim assessment
(f) migrants (lost to follow-up)

(c), (e) and (f) are deviations from protocol; (d) is a deviation from protocol in a fixed-dose clinical trial, but not in a variable-dose study

the pharmacological activity of the drug or about the therapeutic value of a specific modality of treatment. Such studies require quite rigid scientific control, with the treatment groups differing only in the specific factor of interest. It can be appreciated that while explanatory studies are necessary for the development of pharmacological treatments, the search for active subcomponents of therapy, and for the testing of scientific theories, they provide little information about the benefits and problems of treatment in routine clinical use.

Pragmatic trials are designed to answer questions of practical importance in the treatment of patients; they compare the *policy* of giving one treatment with the policy of giving another by analysing the trial data on the basis of the 'intention to treat', that is, all randomised patients are followed up and assessed as required by the protocol *irrespective* of changes in, or non-compliance with, the prescribed treatment. There appears little point in using placebo controls in such trials since placebo by itself is not a form of treatment prescribed in routine clinical use. However, with psychiatric illnesses it is frequently difficult to obtain objective response criteria when treatment is known, particularly when patients are followed up through interim assessments, so some form of placebo control may be necessary to enable objective assessment of outcome. At the same time, the difficulties with using placebos should not be underestimated given that most active treatments are associated with well recognised side-effects.

A major problem with many clinical trials in psychiatry is that they are conceived and designed as explanatory studies aimed at answering a question of scientific importance (perhaps mainly of academic interest) but in a clinical environment where rigid control cannot be maintained. Protocol deviations, as exemplified by Fig. 2.8, mean that at the end of the study the investigator is faced by a difficult choice: either to abandon those patients who do not conform to the protocol and attempt an explanatory analysis of those who do (a procedure fraught with selection bias), or to abandon the explanatory analysis (and the question of scientific importance) by using all the available data in a pragmatic analysis, which attempts to answer a question of clinical relevance. The design as an explanatory study may vitiate and frustrate this process.

The problem can be resolved only partially. The investigators must summarise *all* known protocol deviations in their report and present an initial analysis of all trial entrants as randomised. Subsequent analyses on subgroups of patients may be conducted and reported but there must be clear statements about which patients and which data were excluded, so that critical readers can form opinions about the validity of the investigators' claims.

Missing data

Apart from deviations from protocol that arise from known changes in treatments and dosages, as well as non-compliance, it should be anticipated that patients may default follow-up assessment, resulting in missing data on treatment and clinical status. Such missing data must be anticipated at the stage of trial design, eliminated as far as possible by efficient follow-up procedures and catered for in the analysis by some method of estimation, for example using the last value carried forward. More than a small amount of missing data suggests that the trial design or the instruments chosen for assessment are inadequate.

There is a tendency in psychiatric studies to attempt quite frequent follow-up, often with batteries of psychometric tests and other assessments. Yet the best tests available will be useless if patients cannot be persuaded to turn up for interview, or decline to undertake them. One solution lies in simplicity: increase the sample size, reduce the number of interim assessments (even to none!), and use a simple measure of response.

Choice of treatments

It is important to heed Bradford Hill's description quoted at the beginning of the chapter and emphasise that clinical trials are "applicable with . . . any treatment". Some may think of the clinical trial solely as a research vehicle for the licensing of new pharmaceutical products. This could not be further from the truth. Any treatment whether drug, electroconvulsive therapy (ECT), counselling, psychotherapy, diet, intensity of follow-up, referral practice, even complementary therapy is amenable to comparative evaluation by a clinical trial. Some argue vigorously that it is important to test scientific theories by looking contemporaneously at different presentations of the same drug, or at (side-chain) modifications of a proven agent, or at different forms of psychotherapy in explanatory trials. So be it, but in phase III studies it is generally worthwhile maximising the difference between the forms of treatment under study and thus answering a question of direct clinical relevance. For example it is feasible to conduct a pragmatic trial comparing a policy of drug treatment (the exact choice left to each psychiatrist), a policy of ECT (again the specific form left to each psychiatrist) and a policy of psychotherapy (determined by the psychiatrists).

Power and confidence

Many clinical trials and certainly most of those conducted in psychiatry give little if any consideration to the determination of the sample size at the design stage (Freiman *et al*, 1978). Medical journals continue to publish useless studies with too few patients in each treatment group, without any indication of the implication of such sample sizes for the precision of the estimated differences between treatments. Thus one of the most important aspects of clinical trial design, namely the choice of sample size, is based not on some rational calculation but is left irresponsibly to be determined by the numbers of patients available at some clinic or hospital or who can be studied within some convenient set period. One approach to the rational determination of sample size is via the concept of statistical power, which, although not a panacea for subjectivity, should prevent total wastage of valuable patient resources in unethical studies.

As an introduction to this concept we consider as before a parallel group study with two treatment groups, amitriptyline and mianserin, in patients with a history of affective illness, suffering from a current episode of depression. We will assume that response to treatment is measured by a dichotomous variable categorised as 'response' or 'no response' on the basis of a clinical rating performed four weeks after randomisation and treatment. It is also assumed from the results of previous studies that about 30% of patients will be judged to respond on this measure. We wish to design a clinical trial that will detect at least a 15% difference in response between the treatments. By this we mean, that if the difference in response rates is really as large as 15%, then a (two-tailed) statistical test of the difference in response rates actually observed in the trial will be significant at the 5% level of probability (that is $P<0.05$). In practice, as a result of sampling and response variation, we can never be absolutely certain that the observed difference in response rates will be significant at $P = 0.05$ even if there really is a 15% difference in efficacy. If we imagine that there is no difference in efficacy but the trial indicates a statistically significant difference we will have obtained a false positive result and committed a type I error, α; on the other hand if there really is a difference in efficacy of at least 15% and the difference in the trial is statistically not significant (at $P = 0.05$) then we have obtained a false negative result and committed a type II error, β. The best we can achieve in designing the trial is to choose the sample size in such a way that we impose reasonable limits on the two types of error.

The type I error rate α is equal to the level of probability chosen for declaring the difference between response rates significant; in this example α is 0.05 or 5%. So there is one chance in 20 of getting a false positive result. If this is considered unacceptable then we could lower the type I error rate by reducing the P value for significance to 0.01, or 1%. The type II error rate β is more difficult to calculate, being dependent upon the type I error, α, the sample size and the difference in efficacy to be detected. In practice, instead of working directly with β, statisticians think in terms of $1-\beta$ or $100(1-\beta)$, which is called the power or sensitivity of the trial. In our example, it is the probability that the outcome of the trial will be statistically significant at $P = 0.05$, given that there is at least a 15% difference in response rates. For most statistical tests, tables are available that show the power of the test to detect specified differences for a given α and sample size, as well as tables that show the required sample size to achieve selected power for specified differences and given α (Cohen, 1977; Lachin, 1981; Donner, 1984; Machin & Campbell, 1987). Table 2.3 is an extract chosen to illustrate the example we are considering. In designing a clinical trial, we should select the power $1-\beta$ to be at least 0.80, so that there is a chance of one in five or less of missing an important difference between treatments. (The survey by Freiman *et al* (1978) demonstrates that the power of published studies to detect substantial differences is often very low.) It can be seen from Table 2.3 that with $\alpha = 0.05$, $\beta = 0.20$, power = $1-\beta = 1 - 0.20 = 0.80$, we require about 160 patients per treatment group. If we decide to increase the power to 90%, giving a chance of one in ten of a false negative result, then 220 patients per treatment group are required; if in addition, α is reduced to 0.01 (i.e. 1%) then 240 patients per treatment group are required

TABLE 2.3
Numbers of patients required in each of two groups to detect changes in response rates of 10%, 15% and 20% when the smaller response rate is 30% at a significance level,
$\alpha = 0.05$ *(two-tailed)*

Power	Difference in response rates		
(%)	10%	15%	20%
20	55	25	15
30	95	40	25
40	130	60	35
50	175	80	50
60	220	100	60
70	280	125	75
80	360	160	95
90	480	220	125

Example: to have 80% power of detecting a change in response rates from 30% to 45% requires 160 patients *in each group.*

for a power of 80%, and 305 patients per treatment group for a power of 90% (not shown in Table 2.3). If we are interested in detecting smaller differences in response rates, say of the order of 10%, then we require correspondingly larger sample sizes. (With $\alpha = 0.05$ and power 80% we need 360 patients, and with power 90%, we require 480 patients in each treatment group.) Compare these with the actual sizes of published trials!

Besides calculating the sample sizes necessary to achieve given type I and type II error rates, for specific response rates and differences between them at the design stage, we can also investigate the power of a given clinical trial to detect specific differences once it is completed. Such calculations are important in interpreting non-significant results. In Table 2.4 we show some hypothetical results from a clinical trial. Note that the response rate in the amitriptyline group is in line with the expected response rate of 30% while that in the mianserin group is 50%, a difference between treatments of 20%. From Table 2.3 we can see that with 40 patients per group the trial has a power of just over 40% to detect a 20% difference in response rates given that such a difference exists. So the non-significant χ^2 test is no surprise! With half this number of patients and similar response rates the situation is rather worse; now there is only about 25% power of detecting a 20% difference. Indeed, there is 50% power (an even chance!) of detecting a difference of 30% in response rates given that such a difference exists. With double the numbers of patients, that is 80 per treatment group, we have over 70% chance of detecting a real difference of 20%.

But how should we interpret the results in Table 2.4(a), (b) and (c)? The temptation, indeed the usual practice, is to interpret a non-significant test ('NS') as synonymous with no treatment difference. This is utterly fallacious! Instead of merely reporting the results of tests of statistical significance, we need to report the precision of our estimate of the difference in response rates for the two treatments. This can be done by a 95% confidence limit

TABLE 2.4
Hypothetical results from a clinical trial of the comparative efficacy of amitriptyline and mianserin

		Amitriptyline	Mianserin	Total
(a)	Response	12	20	32
	No response	28	20	48
	Total	40	40	80
	$\chi^2 = 3.3$, d.f. = 1, $P > 0.05$			
(b)	Response	6	10	16
	No response	14	10	24
	Total	20	20	40
	$\chi^2 = 1.7$, d.f. = 1, $P > 0.05$			
(c)	Response	24	40	64
	No response	56	40	96
	Total	80	80	160
	$\chi^2 = 6.7$, d.f. = 1, $P < 0.01$			

Response rates in amitriptyline and mianserin groups are 30% and 50% respectively.
d.f. = degrees of freedom; χ^2 not corrected for continuity.

for the difference (Gardner & Altman, 1986). We note from Table 2.4 that the differences between response rates are always 50–30% or 20%; the 95% confidence limits for this difference are −9% and 50% for Table 2.4(b), −1% and 41% for Table 2.4(a), and 5% and 35% for Table 2.4(c). The lesson is obvious. As the sample size increases, the precision of the estimate of the difference between treatments increases – the width of the 95% confidence interval decreases from 59%, through 42% to 30%. With small numbers our estimates of the difference between treatments are very imprecise, and certainly insufficient to guide clinical practice.

Although the example above is centred on a dichotomous response variable, similar calculations can be performed for a continuous variable. The only complication is that we need to have an estimate of the variation in response. Let us assume that in the clinical trial in our example above, the Hamilton Rating Scale for Depression (HRSD) is used to assess affective status. We can assume that randomisation will balance the distribution of baseline Hamilton scores in the two treatment groups and so use the scores after four weeks as our measure of response. The mean scores in the two groups at four weeks will then be compared with a *t*-test. Assume that we require an 80% power to detect a difference of six points on the HRSD between treatment groups at $P = 0.05$ (smaller differences will be hard work to detect and may not be clinically impressive). To carry out our sample size calculation we need an estimate of the standard deviation of the distribution of HRSD scores at four weeks. This information should be available from previous studies but we will assume estimates of 4, 6 and 8 units. Dividing the required difference of 6 units by the standard deviation provides a standardised difference or an effect size (ES); here the effect sizes are 1.5, 1.0 and 0.75 respectively. Tables of the numbers of patients to achieve given power for set values of α and different values of the effect size are available (Cohen, 1977). These indicate that we need group sizes of about 8, 17 and 30, for the three situations to achieve 80% power and 10, 22 and 40 for 90% power. In fact these sample sizes should be regarded with some caution since in practice HRSD scores at four weeks may not be normally distributed thus invalidating direct application of the *t*-test to the raw scores. A square-root transformation may be necessary. In addition HRSD scores may also be obtained at interim assessments say, at weeks 1, 2 and 3, in which case the analysis will become a repeated measures analysis of variance with treatment differences assessed from the test for interaction effects with a consequent increase in power.

With multiple-response variables the probability of a false positive result (type I error) will be increased. So some adjustment for multiple comparisons will be necessary to retain an overall type I error rate α of about 5%. This will inflate the necessary sample size. One approach, known as the Bonferroni method (Godfrey, 1985), is to divide the overall type I error rate, α, by the number of response variables and use the resultant P value as the level of probability for declaring statistical significance. For example with five response variables and $\alpha = 0.05$ (overall type I error rate), each response variable would be assessed using $P = 0.05/5 = 0.01$. Apart from allowance for multiple comparisons, the sample size derived from a power calculation at the design stage should be increased by about 10% (not more) to account for loss to follow-up.

Analysis

We have commented already on some of the important issues in the analysis of data collected during clinical trials; here we reiterate these and comment briefly on a few more, but for a full discussion the reader is referred to the list of further reading cited at the end of this chapter.

The first point to re-emphasise is that to carry out a sensible and informative analysis it is necessary to have a sufficient quantity of high-quality data. No amount of skillful adjustment or manipulation will compensate for more than a small amount of missing information. In psychiatric studies in particular, there is a tendency to collect far more data than can be justified by the sample size. Investigators should elect at the design stage to ask of every single item of information that it is intended to seek, whether it is essential; the objective should be to eliminate at least 50% of it. During the trial itself, there must be determined efforts to obtain the information required; there is no excuse for more than a tiny number of missing values on baseline variables, whereas missing values on response variables indicate that an alternative method of assessment is required. The first analysis conducted and reported should include *all* randomised patients, and should reflect (at least initially) all features of the design including pre-stratification. Adjustment of the response variables for differences between treatment groups on distributions of baseline variables (post-stratification) should be made *if* such adjustment is considered important. The baseline variables for which to adjust should not be chosen on the basis of statistical significance tests comparing randomised groups; such tests are uninformative (Altman, 1985).

When further analyses are reported it must be clear to the reader exactly which patients have been excluded and why. Treatment differences should be summarised not just by the results of statistical significance tests but in terms of 95% confidence limits for the difference. The power of the clinical trial to detect specified differences between treatment groups should be stated.

In many clinical trials subjects are categorised as responders or non-responders, followed by attempts at analysis of baseline variables to distinguish one group from the other. Few clinical trials are sufficiently large to warrant such abuse and the practice should be abandoned except perhaps within the context of a meta-analysis (National Heart, Lung and Blood Institute & National Cancer Institute, 1987).

Conclusion

The psychiatrist who wishes to conduct a clinical trial should seek advice from at least three experts: first, from a psychiatrist who has performed a clinical trial and can anticipate many of the clinical problems; second, from a physician with experience of clinical trials in another medical discipline who can view the trial within the wider context of medicine; and finally, from a medical statistician (with some knowledge of psychiatry) who can tackle the problems of design and sample size. (Finding one may not be easy but they are around – see for example Committee of Professors of Statistics in the United Kingdom and Ireland (1987) and Agha (1988)). To those who wish to proceed, it is hoped that these notes and the references at the end of the chapter will prove useful.

Appendix: Computer packages and guides

Chapter 13 deals with the use of computers in psychiatric research. More detailed information on computer packages and databases is available from computer centres at most universities throughout the UK, USA and Europe. Potential users are strongly advised to consult local experts before proceeding. The manuals are obtainable through bookshops, or directly from software distributors.

BMDP

BMDP Statistical Software. W. J. Dixon (Chief Editor). University of California Press, Berkeley, 1985.

SAS

SAS User's Guide: Basics. Version 5 Edition, SAS Institute Inc., Cary, NC, 1985.
SAS User's Guide: Statistics. Version 5 Edition, SAS Institute Inc., Cary, NC, 1985.

SPSS

SPSSX User's Guide. 3rd Edition. SPSS Inc., McGraw-Hill, New York, 1988.
Norusis, M. J. SPSSX: Introductory Statistics Guide, SPSS Inc., McGraw-Hill, New York, 1983.
Norusis, M. J. SPSSX: Advanced Statistics Guide, SPSS Inc., McGraw-Hill, New York, 1985.

References

ALTMAN, D. G. (1985) Comparability of randomized groups. *Statistician*, **34**, 125–136.
AGHA, W. M. (1988) *Directory of Academic Statisticians in Polytechnics and Similar Institutions*. Dr W. M. Agha, School of Mathematics, Statistics and Computing, Thames Polytechnic, London SE18 6PF.
ARMITAGE, P. (1975) *Sequential Medical Trials* (2nd edn). Oxford: Blackwell.
BAINES, S., SAXBY, P. & EHLERT, K. (1987) Reality orientation and reminiscence therapy: a controlled crossover study of elderly confused people. *British Journal of Psychiatry*, **151**, 222–231.
BLACKWELL, B. & SHEPHERD, M. (1967) Early evaluation of psychotic drugs in man: a trial that failed. *Lancet*, *ii*, 810–822.
BUTLER, G., CULINGTON, A., HIBBERT, G., *et al* (1987) Anxiety management for persistent generalised anxiety. *British Journal of Psychiatry*, **151**, 535–542.
BUYSE, M. E., STAQUET, M. J. & SYLVESTER, R. J. (eds) (1984) *Cancer Clinical Trials: Methods and Practice*. Oxford: Oxford University Press.
COHEN, J. (1977) *Statistical Power Analysis for the Behavioural Sciences* (2nd edn). New York: Academic Press.
COMMITTEE OF PROFESSORS OF STATISTICS IN THE UNITED KINDGOM AND IRELAND (1987) *Directory of Academic Statisticians*. Ed. and available from Professor R. M. Loynes, Department of Probability and Statistics, University of Sheffield, Sheffield S3 7RH.
COOK, C. C. H., SCANNELL, T. D. & LIPSEDGE, M. S. (1988) Another trial that failed. *Lancet*, *i*, 524–525.
CORNEY, R. H. (1987) Marital problems and treatment outcome in depressed women: a clinical trial of social work and intervention. *British Journal of Psychiatry*, **151**, 652–659.
DONNER, A. (1984) Approaches to sample size estimation in the design of clinical trials – a review. *Statistics in Medicine*, **3**, 199–214.
FREELY, M., CALVERT, R. & GIBSON, J. (1982) Chobazam in catamenial epilepsy: a model for evaluating anti-convulsants. *Lancet*, *ii*, 71–73.
FREIMAN, J. A., CHALMERS, T. C., SMITH, H., *et al* (1978) The importance of beta, the type II error and sample size in the design and interpretation of the randomized control trial. Survey of 71 'negative' trials. *New England Journal of Medicine*, **299**, 690–694.
GARDNER, M. J. & ALTMAN, D. G. (1986) Confidence intervals rather than P-values: estimation rather than hypothesis testing. *British Medical Journal*, **292**, 746–750.
GLEN, A. I. M., JOHNSON, A. L. & SHEPHERD, M. (1984) Continuation therapy with lithium and amitriptyline in unipolar depressive illness: a randomized, double-blind, controlled trial. *Psychological Medicine*, **14**, 37–50.
GODFREY, K. (1985) Comparing the means of several groups. *New England Journal of Medicine*, **313**, 1450–1456.
GORE, S. M. (1981*a*) Assessing clinical trials – record sheets. *British Medical Journal*, **283**, 296–298.

—— (1981*b*) Assessing clinical trials – restricted randomization. *British Medical Journal*, **282**, 2114–2117.
HAMPTON, J. R. (1981) Presentation and analysis of the results of clinical trials in cardiovascular disease. *British Medical Journal*, **282**, 1371–1373.
HILL, A. B. (1955) *Introduction to Medical Statistics* (5th edn). London: Lancet.
HILLS, M. & ARMITAGE, P. (1979) The two-period crossover clinical trial. *British Journal of Clinical Pharmacology*, **8**, 7–20.
JOHNSON, D. A. W., LUDLOW, J. M., STREET, K., *et al* (1987) Double-blind comparison of half-dose and standard-dose flupenthixol decanoate in the maintenance treatment of stabilised outpatients with schizophrenia. *British Journal of Psychiatry*, **151**, 634–638.
JOYCE, C. R. B. & WELLDON, R. M. C. (1965) The objective efficacy of prayer: a double-blind clinical trial. *Journal of Chronic Diseases*, **18**, 367–377.
LACHIN, J. M. (1981) Introduction to sample size determination and power analysis for clinical trials. *Controlled Clinical Trials*, **2**, 93–113.
MACHIN, D. & CAMPBELL, M. J. (1987) *Statistical Tables for the Design of Clinical Trials*. Oxford: Blackwell.
MEINERT, C. L. (1986) *Clinical Trials: Design, Conduct and Analysis*. Oxford: Oxford University Press.
MILLAR, K. (1983) Clinical trial design: the neglected problem of asymmetrical transfer in crossover trials. *Psychological Medicine*, **13**, 867–873.
NATIONAL HEART, LUNG AND BLOOD INSTITUTE & NATIONAL CANCER INSTITUTE (1987) Proceedings of Methodologic Issues in Overviews of Randomized Clinical Trials Workshop. *Statistics in Medicine*, **6**, 217–409.
POCOCK, S. J. (1978) The size of cancer clinical trials and stopping rules. *British Journal of Cancer*, **38**, 757–766.
VALLEJO, J., GASTO, C., CATALAN, R., *et al* (1987) Double-blind study of imipramine versus phenelzine in melancholia and dysthymic disorders. *British Journal of Psychiatry*, **151**, 639–642.
WHITE, S. J. & FREEDMAN, L. S. (1978) Allocation of patients to treatment groups in a controlled clinical study. *British Journal of Cancer*, **37**, 434–447.
WRIGHT, P. & HAYBITTLE, J. (1979) Design of forms for clinical trials. *British Medical Journal*, *ii*, 529–530; 590–592; 650–651.

Further reading

BUNCHER, C. P. & TSAY, T. Y. (eds) (1981) *Statistics in the Pharmaceutical Industry*. Basel: Dekker.
CHALMERS, T. C., SMITH, H., BLACKBURN, B., *et al* (1981) A method of assessing the quality of a randomised clinical trial. *Controlled Clinical Trials*, **2**, 31–49.
CHAPUT DE TONGE, D. M. (1977) Aide-mémoire for preparing clinical trial protocols. *British Medical Journal*, *i*, 1323–1324.
FRIEDMAN, L. M., FURBERG, C. D. & DEMETS, D. L. (1981) *Fundamentals of Clinical Trials*. Bristol: Wright.
GOOD, C. S. (ed.) (1976) *The Principles and Practice of Clinical Trials*. Edinburgh: Churchill Livingstone.
GORE, S. M. & ALTMAN, D. G. (1982) *Statistics in Practice*. London: British Medical Association.
JOHNSON, F. N. & JOHNSON, S. (eds) (1977) *Clinical Trials*. Oxford: Blackwell.
MEINERT, C. L. (1986) *Clinical Trials: Design, Conduct and Analysis*. Oxford: Oxford University Press.
MOSTELLER, F., GILBERT, J. P. & MCPEEK, B. (1980) Reporting standards and research strategies for controlled trials. *Controlled Clinical Trials*, **1**, 37–58.
PETO, R., PIKE, M. C., ARMITAGE, P., *et al* (1976, 1977) Design and analysis of randomized clinical trials requiring prolonged observation of each patient. I. Introduction and design. II. Analysis and examples. *British Journal of Cancer*, **34**, 585–618; **35**, 1–39.
POCOCK, S. J. (1983) *Clinical Trials: a Practical Approach*. Chichester: Wiley.
SHAPIRO, S. H. & LOUIS, T. A. (eds) (1983) *Clinical Trials – Issues and Approaches*. Basel: Dekker.
TYGSTRUP, N., LACHIN, J. M. & JUHL, E. (1982) *The Randomized Clinical Trial and Therapeutic Decisions*. New York: Dekker.

3 Research methods appropriate to biological psychiatry

EVE JOHNSTONE and
M. TIMOTHY LAMBERT

Biological psychiatry is concerned with the idea that psychiatric disorders are associated with demonstrable anatomical or physiological abnormalities. These abnormalities may provide evidence of the basis of the disorder (e.g. the pathology of neurosyphilis) or they may be epiphenomena, which may be used as measures of severity (e.g. heart rate or measures of sweating in anxiety). The anatomy or physiology in which dysfunction is sought is generally, although not exclusively, that of the nervous system.

In psychiatric research the biological variables that are considered to be indications of structural or functional abnormality in the nervous system are related to clinical variables, generally either diagnostic assessments or indices of severity. It is important to remember that the strength of any chain of research is in its weakest link, and sophisticated chemistry cannot make up for careless or ill thought out clinical methods. Diagnostic methods must be clear cut and well described. It is important to match the control sample with the patient sample as closely as possible for age, sex and other demographic variables, but it is also necessary to consider the possibility of there being some difference between patients and controls other than the diagnosis in question.

There are many examples in the literature of apparent biological correlates of psychiatric disorders which have appeared convincing and important at one time but which have not been sustained by subsequent experiments and have faded away "like elephants' footprints in the mud" (*Lancet*, 1978). Quite frequently they have faded away because of patient/control differences that were not taken into account in the initial experiments. Platelet monoamine oxidase activity was reported to be significantly reduced in schizophrenic patients compared with controls (Murphy & Wyatt, 1972). This topic received extensive further study, some investigations confirming the original findings and others not, but it was later shown that there are slow effects of neuroleptics upon the activity of this enzyme which could account for the reduction (Owen *et al*, 1981). It has been claimed that non-suppression of cortisol following dexamethasone may be used as a diagnostic test for depression of the endogenous type (Carroll *et al*, 1980). This finding has been replicated by some and not by others and non-suppression certainly occurs in a variety of other psychiatric disorders (Braddock, 1986) and in association with weight loss in anorexics, in normal or obese subjects and depressed patients (Berger *et al*, 1983). In a study of ventricular : brain ratio (VBR) in manic–depressive patients compared with that in neurotic patients significant differences were not established, but 19% of the manic–depressive patients had VBRs more than two standard deviations above the neurotic mean (Johnstone *et al*, 1986*b*). Search for correlates of ventricular enlargement revealed that five of the patients had a history of treated thyroid deficiency and the VBR of the hypothyroid patients was significantly greater than that of the remainder. Otherwise correlates were not found.

Clearly therefore, in diagnosis-related research, accuracy of psychiatric diagnosis is not the only important clinical issue. It is always wise to take a detailed history of drug ingestion and to establish an accurate picture of the present state of health and past medical history of both patients and controls. One of the difficulties of encouraging recruitment of controls from among departmental staff is that they may not consider it appropriate to give an accurate account of family history of mental illness, drug and alcohol ingestion and indeed their own past health. If possible it is best to avoid placing colleagues in this difficult position. Experience shows the advisability of close documentation of all subjects in research projects and of keeping the data. Even though some of it may not seem relevant at the time, it may help with questions raised later; so too may careful clinical descriptions of the patients. Apart from their value in relation to a particular study these are likely to be helpful to later investigators and indeed the greatest benefits from such descriptions may not be derived until after the patient's death. Clinicians involved in post-mortem work often rely at least in part on clinical notes written decades previously. Those which quote what the patient actually said are much more useful than those which describe the presence or absence of various phenomena in general terms.

Studies in which repeated measures of a biological variable are related to a series of assessments of symptom severity in patients whose condition is changing are often conducted in association with treatment trials. It is useful in these circumstances to be able to separate the effects of a treatment from those of change in the condition it is used to treat, and this can be done in the context of controlled clinical trials. It is usual to find significant improvements in placebo groups as a whole in such studies and very substantial improvements in a few patients.

Non-clinical variables examined in relation to biological psychiatry may be classified as follows.

(a) Disorders of function of the central nervous system (CNS)
(b) Disorders of structure of the CNS
(c) Genetic aspects
(d) Other aspects

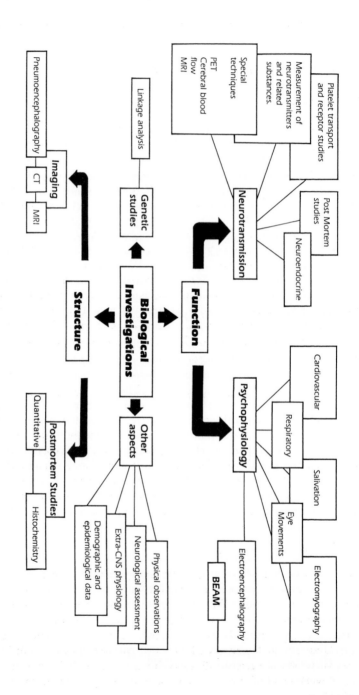

Fig. 3.1 Classification of non-clinical variables used in relation to biological psychiatry

A subclassification in relation to these headings is suggested in Fig.
3.1

Disorders of function of the CNS

Neurotransmission

Largely based on psychopharmacological findings, hypotheses relating
serious psychiatric disorders to neurotransmission have been derived in the
last 20 years and have received much support (noradrenaline and
5-hydroxytryptamine for affective disorders (Schildkraut, 1965; Lapin &
Oxenkrug, 1969); dopamine for schizophrenia (Snyder *et al*, 1974); acetyl
choline for dementing illness (Bowen *et al*, 1976)). Considerable research
effort has been expended upon the study of these classic neurotransmitters
and there is a good deal of evidence that they are related to psychiatric
disease, but much remains to be discovered. In recent years evidence has
accumulated to show that other substances, in particular peptides, are present
in the nervous system and that these may possess neurotransmitter/modulator
properties (for a review see Roberts *et al*, 1984). Hypotheses that psychiatric
disorders are associated with altered availability or function of
neurotransmitters at certain sites in the brain cannot be directly tested in
human subjects during life. Various indirect measures may however be
used.

Measures of substances related to neurotransmitters in body fluids

It is possible to examine the body fluids (e.g. urine, blood, cerebrospinal
fluid) for neurotransmitters, their precursors and metabolites and substances
directly related to them. This approach was particularly applied to
catecholamine and indolealkylamine pathways in relation to affective illness
(for review see Johnstone, 1982). Useful information has been derived from
these indirect methods, although they are perhaps less fashionable than they
were and have been to some extent replaced by other areas of investigation.

Platelet transport and receptor sites

One such area is the study of platelet transport and receptor sites. Blood
platelets possess monoamine oxidase activity, an active transport process
for 5-hydroxytryptamine (5HT) and the presence of binding sites for α- and
β-adrenoreceptor ligands, 5HT ligands and ^{3}H-imipramine has been
established. Differences between patients (mainly with depression) and
controls have been demonstrated for several of these measures but findings
vary (for review see *Lancet*, 1982; Wood & Coppen, 1985) and this is an
area of work in which findings may be affected by previous psychotropic
medication.

Neuroendocrine methods

Neuropharmacological studies allied with histochemical and immuno-fluorescence techniques have established that neurotransmitters play a crucial role in the modulation of anterior pituitary hormones through an action on the hypothalamic hypophysiotropic neurons (Fuxe & Hokfelt, 1969). Because of the evidence relating schizophrenia to dopaminergic mechanisms (Snyder *et al*, 1974) prolactin has been the most widely studied, in view of the direct nature of the control of secretion of this hormone by dopamine (Ben-Jonathan *et al*, 1977). Growth hormone (GH), luteinising hormone (LH), follicle-stimulating hormone (FSH) and adrenocorticotrophic hormone (ACTH) have also been studied in relation to psychiatric disease (for review see Johnstone & Ferrier, 1981).

Anterior pituitary hormone secretion (APHS) is of course affected by the administration of psychotropic drugs, and prolactin (PRL) levels are used as a measure of the efficacy of the dopaminergic blockade induced by neuroleptic drugs, but APHS may vary in relation to a variety of other factors: for example LH, FSH, ACTH, and GH have markedly episodic secretory patterns; LH, FSH, and PRL secretion varies considerably in relation to the state of maturity of the individual and with the menstrual cycle (Yen, 1977); and PRL, ACTH, and GH have sleep-related secretions which may respond differently to pharmacological stimuli (Rubin, 1977). Feedback effects from target-organ hormone secretion are of major importance to APHS, and non-specific stimuli may be the important determinant of APHS at the time of the study, for example stress on PRL and ACTH, nutritional status on LH and glucose intake on GH (Noel *et al*, 1972; Himsworth *et al*, 1972; Strain & Strain, 1978). Apart from direct measures of hormone levels, functional tests like dexamethasone suppression (Carroll *et al*, 1981), growth hormone and prolactin responses to apomorphine and growth hormone responses to adrenoreceptor blockers (for review see Checkley, 1980; Johnstone & Ferrier, 1981) are used and these are relevant to affective as well as schizophrenic disorders.

Post-mortem techniques

It is possible to analyse post-mortem brain tissue for monoamines, related substances and relevant enzymes. This area of work has greatly illuminated the biological basis of Parkinsonism (Hornykiewicz, 1963), Huntington's chorea (Bird & Iversen, 1974) and senile dementia (Bowen *et al*, 1976). These are conditions which progress until the point of death and although the terminal state and final cause of death has to be considered in relation to this work, as discussed by Bird & Stokes (1982) with reference to Huntington's chorea, there is no real doubt that the disorder diagnosed in life was still present when the patient died. The position is different in affective illness which relapses and remits during life, and however severe it has been at times during life, that patient may die with a normal mental state. The brains of patients committing suicide have been used in the study of monoamine metabolites in relation to depression (Shaw *et al*, 1967; Bourne *et al*, 1968; Pare *et al*, 1969), but the results are not consistent (Johnstone, 1982) and to what extent this inconsistency may relate to the clinical differences which are likely to have operated cannot be established.

Dopamine, its metabolites and related enzymes have been measured in brains from schizophrenic patients and the results have in general shown little consistent evidence of disturbance (for review see Owen *et al*, 1985; Costall & Naylor 1986) but effects of drugs have to be taken into account. Limitations on post-mortem work in schizophrenia are imposed by the fact that the brains are usually obtained many decades after the onset of the disorder and when the positive phenomena (for which the evidence of the involvement of dopaminergic mechanisms is strongest) may have long ceased to be evident, and these limitations should not be ignored. These problems are also applicable to the interpretation of studies of schizophrenic brain using receptor-labelling assays to determine the nature and number of dopamine receptors. Owen *et al* (1978) reported an increase in D_2 receptors in schizophrenic brain. Others have also found this result (for review see Costall & Naylor, 1986) but it is claimed that it is possible that these findings are partly due to previous drug treatment. This is unlikely to explain all the results (Owen *et al*, 1985) but continued exploration of this field is limited by the great difficulty of obtaining brains from patients who are known to have suffered from schizophrenia and who have not had neuroleptic drugs. Immunocytochemistry is used to examine brain tissue for peptides (for review see Roberts *et al*, 1984) but again problems of diagnosis of the patient's clinical state and previous drug treatment have to be considered. It is possible that recently developed special techniques may help to combat some of these problems.

Special techniques

In the last ten years there have been considerable technical advances in imaging methods which have greatly enhanced the opportunities for studying brain function and structure. The techniques most relevant to functional studies are assessments of cerebral blood flow, positron emission tomography (PET) and nuclear magnetic resonance (NMR) spectroscopy. Cerebral blood flow may be studied by radionuclide clearance using ^{133}Xe inhalation (Obrist *et al*, 1975). Oxygen use and glucose metabolism can both be assessed using PET (for review see Frackowiak, 1986) and these techniques have been used to investigate organic and functional psychoses. In addition it is possible to use emission tomography to trace gamma-emitting ligands for particular receptors in the brain. This has been done using ^{77}Br-spiperone (Crawley *et al*, 1986), a ligand for D_2 receptors, and the results offer some support for there being greater receptor activity in untreated schizophrenic patients than in controls. NMR spectroscopy has the potential of providing a non-invasive analytic tool for quantitative measurement *in vivo* of various substances (Hall *et al*, 1986), but this technique is at an early stage of development and localisation remains a difficulty. All of these special techniques for functional studies have yet to realise their full potential. Perusal of some of the work so far conducted underlines the importance of the highest clinical standards being applied to this area (*Lancet*, 1984) as without this, technical sophistication may be wasted.

Psychological studies

These techniques exploit the fact that certain physiological measurements to some extent reflect psychological states or changes. The usefulness of such measures is often limited by the difficulty in separating changes due to psychological activity from those caused by environmental or physical factors, such as exercise and rest, temperature, etc. However, the following measures have been shown to have some relevance to psychiatric research.

Cardiovascular measurements

Of these, the heart rate is the easiest to monitor, using either an electrocardiogram or some form of transducer over an artery or fingertip. These include pressure transducers, photoelectric detectors and microphones. The information thus obtained can be made more useful by converting the pulse signal into electric pulses, the intervals between which can then be displayed on a polygraph or averaged by integrating the pulses. Changes in cardiac rate (Taylor *et al*, 1986) and rhythm (Shear *et al*, 1987) have been studied in patients with panic disorder. Changes in heart rate, along with the changes of skin conductance measures (see below), have been observed during task performance (Frith & Allen, 1983). Intra-arterial catheterisation is used to obtain the very accurate measures of blood flow and blood pressure required for some cardiological purposes, but such techniques are not appropriate in psychophysiological studies, in which surface electrodes and transducers are used to estimate blood flow. For most purposes an adequate intermittent blood pressure reading may be obtained using a sphygmomanometer and arm cuff and, if a systolic pressure alone is adequate, a small cuff on a finger attached to a distal pulse detector may be used.

Penile plethysmography also employs a cuff to measure penile tumescence and this may be used as a measure of male sexual arousal. Thase *et al* (1987) reported a reduction in nocturnal penile tumescence, independent of sleep and disturbance of rapid eye movements (REM) in depressed men.

Respiratory function

Sensitive instruments are available to measure most indices of respiratory function, but these are generally of more interest to the respiratory physician than to the psychiatrist. However, measurements of respiratory rate may be relevant and can be used in conjunction with cardiovascular measures.

Salivation

The estimation of salivation has been used in the study of depressed patients, and under these circumstances whole-mouth salivation as opposed to individual-gland salivation is more relevant. This is achieved using pre-weighed dental rolls which are left in the mouth for a standard time, and then weighed (Peck, 1959).

Skin conductance

The most commonly used measure is the galvanic skin response (GSR), in which the rapid response to a stimulus indicates an increase in activity of the cell membranes of sweat glands. It is a measure that is sensitive to small changes and serial measurements on the same patients may be useful. Although cheap and easy to use, it is important to minimise error and artefact by using appropriate electrodes in areas of skin that are non-thermoregulatory (e.g. the palms or soles) and with the correct contact medium. The skin conductance orientating response to an irrelevant tone has been used as an index of attention in normal subjects (Frith & Allen, 1983). Abnormalities in skin conductance orientating responses, either failure to respond or failure to habituate, have been reported in some groups of schizophrenics (Gruzelier, 1976), and it has been shown (Frith *et al*, 1979) that in acute schizophrenics failure to habituate to tones before treatment tended to predict a poor response to treatment. It is important when using measurements of electrodermal response to take into account the effect of drug treatment (Johnstone *et al*, 1981; Yannitsi *et al*, 1987).

Electromyography

This technique uses electrode placements on the surface of the skin to measure the activities of the underlying muscle. Such signals, when separated from those generated by purposeful activity, provide an index of emotional arousal. Greden *et al* (1986) have reported differences, using facial electromyography, between depressed patients and normal controls.

Eye movements

Using orbital electrodes, the corneo-retinal potential may be measured and this varies with eye movement; thus the number of movements may be determined. This has been of use in sleep research in which REM and REM latency may be measured (e.g. Zarcone *et al*, 1987). Other studies of eye movements, in particular visual tracking, have been carried out in schizophrenic patients and their relatives, in patients with affective disorders (Holzman *et al*, 1973, 1977), and in psychotic patients with thought disorder (Solomon *et al*, 1987).

Electroencephalography

Electroencephalography (EEG) has been in use for many years as a diagnostic and research tool. In the research context single-channel or two-channel readings may be adequate, and changes in patterns will be more relevant than the clear abnormalities of wave-form that are sought by the clinician. Various electronic methods exist to analyse the data, including wave analysis, broad-band pass filtering, and computer analysis. Ambulatory monitoring allows for continuous single-channel or two-channel recording over a space of many hours. Another technique, based on EEG principles, is that of evoked responses, in which the output, following some discrete stimulus such as sound, light flashes, or electric shock, is recorded and separated from the background activity. EEG monitoring and evoked responses have been used in investigations of sleep, depression (Flor-Henry & Koles, 1980), schizophrenia (Connolly *et al*, 1983a), and dementia (Fenton, 1986; Orwin *et al*, 1986).

A more recent development has been to analyse the signals using a computer, and to display these in a dynamic form on a visual display unit. This is known as brain electrical activity mapping (BEAM) and has been used in the study of schizophrenia (Morihisa *et al*, 1983).

Disorders of structure of the CNS

The post-mortem structure of the brain in psychiatric disorders received much attention at the turn of the century and the introduction of pneumoencephalography in 1919 allowed the possibility of examining the anatomy of the brain in life. Pneumoencephalography is associated with technical problems and there are major ethical difficulties in obtaining control subjects for studies using this technique, although investigations of schizophrenic patients have been conducted (Haug, 1962; Storey, 1966). The use of imaging techniques in the study of structural abnormalities in the brain was greatly enhanced by the invention of computerised tomography (CT) by Hounsfield (1973). This procedure gives clear representation of both the lateral and third ventricles; the measure that has gained widest acceptance in the psychiatric literature is the ventricular:brain ratio (VBR). The technique is non-invasive and has allowed normal controls to be compared with patients and the range of appearances in normal subjects to be related to variables such as age. The first CT scan study in schizophrenia (Johnstone *et al*, 1976) found lateral ventricular area to be increased ($P<0.01$) in a group of chronically institutionalised schizophrenic patients in comparison with an age-matched group of normal controls. Numerous subsequent studies of lateral ventricular size have been conducted, and many but not all have confirmed the finding. This area of work has been well reviewed (Weinberger *et al*, 1983; Dewan *et al*, 1986): it appears that the evidence of reduction of brain substance (particularly a degree of ventricular enlargement) occurs in patients with schizophrenia more often than in controls and is not due to treatment (Owens *et al*, 1985). However, this ventricular enlargement is not a necessary concomitant of schizophrenia, even in its most severe and chronic forms, nor is it sufficient for the development of the disease, as such enlargement has been noted in manic–depressive illness (Rieder *et al*, 1983), and as a reversible phenomenon in alcoholism (Carlen *et al*, 1978), anorexia nervosa (Heinz *et al*, 1977) and possibly in patients dependent on benzodiazepines (Lader *et al*, 1984).

A CT scan gives information about the structure and size of the brain but does not provide any information about any pathological processes which might underlie any structural changes demonstrated. Nuclear magnetic resonance, also known as magnetic resonance imaging (MRI), has the potential of providing at least some such information. MRI provides a high level of contrast between grey and white matter, and this is the basis for the application of this technique in the study of demyelinating disease (Young *et al*, 1981). Oedema and inflammatory changes are also well visualised (Steiner & Bydder, 1984) and a characteristic picture is seen in cases of acute encephalitis. The MRI studies of functional psychosis so far conducted (Johnstone *et al*, 1986a; Andreasen *et al*, 1986) have not shown evidence of pathological changes, but the study of Andreasen *et al* (1986) suggested that there was reduced size of brain and skull in the schizophrenic patients. If indeed skull size is reduced in schizophrenic patients compared with controls, it should be possible to demonstrate this using techniques much simpler than MRI.

The results of CT findings have reawakened interest in the post-mortem studies of the structure and histology of the brain in functional psychosis, principally in schizophrenia. Brown *et al* (1986) have shown that the ventricles (particularly the temporal horn of the lateral ventricle) of brains from schizophrenic patients were larger than those from patients with affective illness and that the brain weights of the schizophrenic patients were less. Stevens (1982) reviewed the histological studies performed up until 1970 and found little agreement. Studies since that time have sometimes described an excess of gliosis but this has not been shown in recent, well controlled studies. Kovelman & Scheibel (1984) found cell disarray at the CA_1–CA_2 interfaces of the pyramidal cell layer in schizophrenics compared with controls, and in a similar comparison Benes *et al* (1986) found a reduction in cortical neuronal density in some layers.

Genetic aspects

The biological, as opposed to epidemiological, basis of genetic studies relies on the concept of genetic linkage. Genes that are located near each other on a chromosome are more likely to be transmitted together than are those that are widely separated. Genes from the same chromosome may be separated during meiosis by a process of cross-over or recombination. For a genetic linkage to be useful, it requires first a clear basis for diagnosis in the subject under study and second a clear marker to which it is proposed genetic linkage occurs. The marker must be specific and reliably detectable in those who carry the gene and its manifestations clearly absent in those who do not. A genetic marker may be physiological, such as blood group or eye colour, or phenothiacarbamide tasting, or may be more directly pin-pointed using a genetic probe, that is, a labelled and identified sequence of DNA that will attach itself to a portion of DNA with the corresponding sequence of bases. These sequences may be specific for particular functions, such as enzyme production, and are known as restriction fragment length polymorphisms (RFLP). The chromosomal material under study is separated into fragments using restriction enzymes. If, using these processes, a large number of polymorphisms can be identified, then their coincident existence in members of a family, some of whose members carry the characteristic or disease under study, may be determined and the likelihood of a genetic linkage between the marker and the condition expressed as a probability (logarithm of odds) score.

It is crucial when contemplating this type of study to be aware of three points.

    (a) In psychiatric research, diagnostic separation is rarely clear cut.

    (b) A clear pedigree, containing not less than two affected and some unaffected relatives, is required. Sequential generations, that is parents and their children, are more useful than siblings, and a pedigree with both is better still.

    (c) Similar clinical syndromes may arise from genetic material located at different parts of the chromosome or on different chromosomes and linked to different markers. It should be remembered that in any individual from a pedigree, the genetic linkage may be demonstrable in the absence of the clinical syndrome, either because other factors play a part in the development of the syndrome, or because the individual has not yet reached the age at which the clinical syndrome may become apparent.

Because of the scarcity of suitable pedigrees for genetic study in psychiatric disorders, it is important that, when such pedigrees are identified, centres investigating the disorder in question should be involved in the research planning.

A major achievement in this field was the identification by Gusella *et al* (1983) of a polymorphic DNA marker that is closely linked to Huntington's disease, and which maps to chromosome 4. The hereditary basis of this disorder is well established, but there has been no method available for identifying affected individuals from those at risk. This has seriously limited the scope of individual and genetic counselling since the clinical syndrome is not generally expressed until after the decision as to whether or not to have children has been made. Clearly the chromosome 4 marker has important clinical implications and also provides the basis for further research to locate the Huntington's gene with greater precision, and to elucidate the mechanisms by which the disease is expressed.

Other disorders that have been subject to this type of genetic research include affective disorder, particularly among the Amish community in North America (Egeland *et al*, 1987) and in an Icelandic pedigree (Hodgkinson *et al*, 1987), schizophrenia (McGuffin *et al*, 1983; Andrew *et al*, 1987), late paraphrenia (Naguib *et al*, 1987), Alzheimer's disease (Renvoize, 1984; Nerl *et al*, 1984) and Parkinson's disease (Nerl *et al*, 1984). Recent work has shown that the genetic defect causing familial Alzheimer's disease maps on chromosome 21 (St George-Hyslop *et al*, 1987), thus providing an explanation for the association between Down's syndrome and this disorder.

Other aspects

Biological psychiatry is concerned with the idea that psychiatric disorders are associated with demonstrable anatomical and physiological abnormality. While in general the measures of anatomical and physiological abnormality that are related to clinical psychiatric assessment are derived from the central nervous system, abnormalities relating to other systems may also be relevant.

Physical observations

Kretschmer (1936) attempted to draw links between body types and personality, and between personality and mental illness. This work has not gained scientific support but some of the terms used (schizoid, pyknic, asthenic) have persisted. Sheldon (1942) also attempted to delineate morphological dimensions and personality types. More sophisticated assessments of physical differences have focused on minor physical anomalies and neurological 'soft signs'. Minor physical anomalies include such features as 'electric' hair, head circumference outside normal range, hypertelorism, low-seated ears, adherent ear lobes, high-steepled palate, curver fifth finger, and long third toe. The Waldrop scale (Waldrop *et al*, 1986) may be used to quantify anomalies, weighting certain features and producing a score. Waldrop *et al* (1986) examined pre-school children and the results suggested an association between high anomaly scores and a tendency to increased aggressiveness, behavioural disturbance and hyperkinesis. Rosenberg & Weller (1973), using the same scale, found a higher incidence of anomalies in boys than girls, and an association between high 'stigmata' scores and early academic failure. A raised incidence of anomalies has been reported in schizophrenics as a group, compared with normal controls (Guy *et al*, 1983) and it has been found that those individuals with a greater number of anomalies tended to have poor pre-morbid adjustment. Green *et al* (1987) reported evidence that early-onset schizophrenia is associated with such anomalies, and it is suggested by both groups of authors that events in the first trimester give rise to CNS vulnerability and a high incidence of anomalies. A raised incidence of anomalies has also been reported in autistic children (Walker, 1977; Campbell *et al*, 1978).

Quitkin *et al* (1976) reported an increased incidence of soft neurological signs in schizophrenics with pre-morbid asociality, and in individuals with emotionally unstable character disorders. In this study the soft-signs inventory included assessment of speech, cranial nerves, peripheral sensation, reflexes, muscle strength, co-ordination, tests of stereognosis, graphaesthesia and simultaneous stimulation (the face–hand test) and of the presence of adventitious overflow movement. This evaluation is similar to that used by Hertzig & Birch (1966, 1968) in their investigations of disturbed adolescents. A raised incidence of such soft signs was also found in a mixed group of young adult psychiatric patients compared with controls in a study by Rochford *et al* (1970), in which it was noted that no neurological abnormalities were found among patients with affective disorder.

Owens & Johnstone (1980) found neurological abnormalities in the majority of over 500 long-term in-patients with schizophrenia. In most patients, not all of whom had received neuroleptic medication, these included 'extrapyramidal' signs, involuntary movement disorders, and disturbances of muscle tone, but in 28 patients neurological abnormalities other than these were found.

Laterality

Cerebral dominance, laterality and handedness have been investigated in a variety of psychiatric disorders. However, the validity of some of the methods used has been questioned by McManus (1983), who emphasises the importance of distinguishing differences in degree of laterality from differences in direction of laterality. Provided no forced change has occurred, handedness may be taken as the hand used for writing (McManus, 1984). A more detailed assessment using a 12-item questionnaire (Annett, 1970) has been used (e.g. Taylor *et al*, 1980).

Evidence supporting an increased frequency of sinistrals and mixed handedness in schizophrenics has been reported (Lishman & McMeekan, 1976; Nasrallah *et al*, 1981) and in these reports handedness is taken to be an indicator of cerebral dominance. Shimizu *et al* (1985) have reported an increased frequency of original left or mixed handedness and of converted right handedness in schizophrenics, compared with healthy students, using a questionnaire. Hauser *et al* (1985) emphasised the importance of sex differences in such studies. Fleminger *et al* (1977), in a study of 800 psychiatric patients and 800 controls, found a higher proportion of fully right-handed subjects among psychotics. Bakan (1971) has suggested that sinistrality may be associated with high-risk birth orders (first born and late born), and hence with pre- or perinatal neurological insult. However, in a series of large studies, using data from the National Child Development Study (NCDS) and examining a wide range of obstetric factors, there was no substantial evidence to relate birth stress and left handedness (McManus, 1981).

A review (Taylor *et al*, 1982) of two studies by Lishman & McMeekan (1976) and Fleminger *et al* (1977) emphasises their discrepant findings, points out the pitfalls of this type of research, and underscores the need for careful separation of diagnostic subgroups, age and sex.

Other investigations of cerebral dominance in relation to psychiatric issues have included EEG (Flor-Henry & Koles, 1980; Connolly *et al*, 1983*b*), measurements of regional cerebral blood flow (Gur *et al*, 1985) and clinical assessment of stroke patients (Robinson *et al*, 1985). A review of laterality investigations (Gruzelier, 1981) examines the techniques used and highlights the difficulties in interpreting the data and the studies drawn from them.

Gastrointestinal studies

Investigations relating to diet with reference to psychiatric disorder have been developed. These include estimation of antibodies to food fractions (Dohan *et al*, 1972), intestinal permeability studies (Bjarnason *et al*, 1983; Wood *et al*, 1987; Lambert *et al*, 1987) and challenge/withdrawal studies (Singh & Kay, 1976; Osborne *et al*, 1982).

Demographic data with biological implications

Epidemiological studies may have considerable relevance to biological research. Studies of the association of psychiatric illnesses and physical disease, such as that described by Baldwin (1979), and of the relationship between seasonality of birth and psychiatric disease (Dalen, 1975; Hare & Walter, 1978) have been conducted. Investigation of the season of birth in schizophrenics, manic–depressives, neurotic depressives, and normal controls has demonstrated a consistent excess of birth in the first quarter of the year for the first two groups (Odegard, 1974; Hare, 1975*a, b*; Odegard, 1974). In addition Hare & Walter (1978) have shown that schizophrenics and manics show a marked seasonal variation in admission to hospital, with a maximum in the summer months, in comparison with non-psychotic patients. Such data have given rise to causal hypotheses concerning breeding patterns (Hare & Walter, 1978) and aetiology (Crow, 1986). This type of research demands very large numbers of patients and careful control for factors such as cultural and occupational norms, availability of hospital beds and patterns of care, as well as diagnostic accuracy.

Conclusions

The biological aspects of psychiatry may be considered as more austere, academic and scientific than other areas of study related to mental disease. This may well be true and yet underlying this area of endeavour there is belief as well as hard fact. The belief is in the idea expressed by our 19th-century predecessors such as Kraepelin (1896) and Clouston (1891) as well as by the ancients (Areteus, 1972–written c. AD 150) that psychiatric illnesses are diseases for which pathological bases will be demonstrated. For many of the conditions with which we are concerned there is still no anatomical or physiological abnormality that is reliably found in those affected with the condition in question and not in other people. The belief that these are biological conditions is still therefore a matter of conviction based upon evidence which is not yet adequate, even though much progress has been made since the days of Kraepelin and Clouston. Hard facts are accumulating, some from sophisticated technological advances, some from careful observation, and some more or less serendipitous, so that it is possible to question the 'functional' basis of at least some of the major disorders with which we are concerned (Tyrer & Mackay, 1986).

References

ANDREASEN, N., NASRALLAH, H. A., DUNN, V., *et al* (1986) Structural abnormalities in the frontal system in schizophrenia. *Archives of General Psychiatry*, **43**, 136–144.

ANDREW, B., WATT, D. C., GILLESPIE, C., *et al* (1987) A study of genetic linkage in schizophrenia. *Psychological Medicine*, **17**, 363–370.

ANNETT, M. (1970) A classification of hand preference by association analysis. *British Journal of Psychiatry*, **61**, 303–321.

ARETEUS, THE CAPPADOCIAN (1972) *The Extant Works*, reprint of 1856 edn (ed. and trans. F. Adams). Boston: Milford House Inc.

BAKAN, P. (1971) Handedness and birth order. *Nature*, **229**, 195.

BALDWIN, J. A. (1979) Schizophrenia and physical disease. *Psychological Medicine*, **9**, 611–618.

BEN-JONATHAN, N., OLIVER, C., WEINER, H. J., *et al* (1977) Dopamine in hypophyseal postal plasma of the rat during the oestrus cycle and throughout pregnancy. *Endocrinology*, **100**, 452–458.

BENES, F. M., DAVIDSON, J. & BIRD, E. D. (1986) Quantitative cytoarchitectural studies of the cerebral cortex of schizophrenics. *Archives of General Psychiatry*, **43**, 31–35.

BERGER, M., PIRKE, K. M., DOERR, P., *et al* (1983) Influence of weight loss on the dexamethasone suppression test. *Archives of General Psychiatry*, **40**, 584–586.

BIRD, E. D. & IVERSEN, L. L. (1974) Huntington's chorea–post-mortem measurement of glutamic acid decarboxylase, choline acetyltransferase and dopamine in basal ganglia. *Brain*, **97**, 457–472.

—— & SPOKES, E. G. S. (1982) Huntington's chorea. In *Disorders of Neurohumoural Transmission* (ed. T. J. Crow). London: Academic Press.

BJARNASON, I., PETERS, T. J. & VEALL, N. (1983) A persistent defect in intestinal permeability in coeliac disease demonstrated by a 51/CrEDTA absorption test. *Lancet*, *i*, 323–325.

BOURNE, H. R., BUNNEY, W. E., COLBURN, R. W., *et al* (1968) Noradrenaline, 5-hydroxytryptamine and 5-hydroxyindoleacetic acid in hindbrains of suicidal patients. *Lancet*, *ii*, 805–808.

BOWEN, D. M., SMITH, C. B., WHITE, P., *et al* (1976) Neurotransmitter-related enzymes and indices of hypoxia in senile dementia and other abiotropies. *Brain*, **99**, 459–496.

BRADDOCK, L. (1986) The dexamethasone suppression test–fact and artefact. *British Journal of Psychiatry*, **148**, 363–374.

BROWN, R., COLTER, N., CORSELLIS, J. A. N., *et al* (1986) Post-mortem evidence of structural brain change in schizophrenia. *Archives of General Psychiatry*, **43**, 36–42.

CAMPBELL, M., GELLAR, B., SMALL, A. M., *et al* (1978) Minor physical anomalies in young psychotic children. *American Journal of Psychiatry*, **135**, 573–575.

CARLEN, P. L., WORTZMAN, G., HOLGATE, R. C., *et al* (1978) Reversible cerebral atrophy in recently abstinent chronic alcoholics measured by computed tomography scans. *Science*, **200**, 1076–1078.

CARROLL, B. J., GREDEN, J. F. & Feinberg, M. (1980) Neuroendocrine disturbances and the diagnosis and aetiology of endogenous depression. *Lancet*, *i*, 321–322.

——, FEINBERG, M., GREDEN, J. F., *et al* (1981) A specific laboratory test for the diagnosis of melancholia. *Archives of General Psychiatry*, **38**, 15–22.

CHECKLEY, S. A. (1980) Neuroendocrine tests of monoamine function in man: a review of basic theory and the application to the study of depressive illness. *Psychological Medicine*, **10**, 35–53.

CLOUSTON, T. S. (1891) *The Neuroses of Development, Being the Morison Lectures of 1890*. Edinburgh: Oliver and Boyd.

CONNOLLY, J. F., GRUZELIER, J. H. & MANCHANDA, R. (1983) Electrocortical and perceptual asymmetries in schizophrenia. In *Laterality and Psychopathology. Developments in Psychiatry*, vol. 6 (eds P. Flor-Henry & J. Gruzelier), pp. 363–378. Amsterdam: Elsevier Science Publishers.

——, ——, ——, *et al* (1983) Visual evoked potentials in schizophrenia. Intensity effects and hemisphere asymmetry. *British Journal of Psychiatry*, **142**, 152–155.

COSTALL, B. & NAYLOR, R. J. (1986) Neurotransmitter hypothesis of schizophrenia. In *The Psychopharmacology of Schizophrenia* (eds P. B. Bradley & S. R. Hirsch). Oxford: Oxford University Press.

CRAWLEY, J. C. W., CROW, T. J., JOHNSTONE, E. C., *et al* (1986) Uptake of [77]Br-spiperone in the striata of schizophrenic patients and controls. *Nuclear Medicine Communications*, **7**, 599–607.

CROW, T. J. (1986) The continuum of psychosis and its implication for structure of the gene. *British Journal of Psychiatry*, **149**, 419–429.

DALEN, P. (1975) *Season of Birth: A Study of Schizophrenic and Other Mental Disorders*. Amsterdam: North Holland.

DEWAN, M. J., PANDURANGI, A. K., LEE, S. H., *et al* (1986) A comprehensive study of chronic schizophrenic patients. *Acta Psychiatrica Scandinavica*, **73**, 152–160.

DOHAN, F. C., MARTIN, L., GRASBERGER, J. C., *et al* (1972) Antibodies to wheat gliadin in blood of psychiatric patients; possible role of emotional factors. *Biological Psychiatry*, **5**, 127–137.

EGELAND, J. A., GERHARD, D. S., PAULS, D. L., *et al* (1987) Bipolar affective disorders linked to DNA markers on chromosome II. *Nature*, **325**, 783–787.

FENTON, G. W. (1986) Electrophysiology of Alzheimer's disease. *British Medical Bulletin*, **42**, 29–33.

FLEMINGER, J. J., DALTON, R. & STANDAGE, K. F. (1977) Handedness in psychiatric patients. *British Journal of Psychiatry*, **131**, 448–452.

FLOR-HENRY, P. & Koles, Z. J. (1980) EEG studies in depression, mania and normals: evidence for partial shifts of laterality in the affective psychoses. *Advances in Biological Psychiatry*, **4**, 21–43.

FRACKOWIAK, R. S. J. (1986) An introduction to positron tomography and its application to clinical investigation. In *New Brain Imaging Techniques and Psychopharmacology*, BAP monograph no. 9 (ed. M.R. Trimble), pp. 25–34. Oxford: Oxford University Press.

FRITH, C. D., STEVENS, M., JOHNSTONE, E. C., *et al* (1979) Skin conductance responsivity during acute episodes of schizophrenia as a predictor of symptomatic improvement. *Psychological Medicine*, **9**, 101–106.
—— & ALLEN, H. A. (1983) The skin conductance orienting response as an index of attention. *Biological Psychology*, **17**, 27–39.
FUXE, K. & HOKFELT, T. (1969) Catecholamines in the hypothalamus and pituitary gland. In *Frontiers in Neuroendocrinology* (eds W. F. Ganarg & L. Martini). New York: Oxford University Press.
GREDEN, J. F., GENERO, N., PRICE, L., *et al* (1986) Facial electromyography in depression. *Archives of General Psychiatry*, **43**, 269–274.
GREEN, M. F., SALZ, P., SOPER, H. V., *et al* (1987) Relationship between physical anomalies and age at onset of schizophrenia. *American Journal of Psychiatry*, **144**, 666–667.
GRUZELIER, J. H. (1976) Clinical attributes of schizophrenic skin conductance responders and non-responders. *Psychological Medicine*, **6**, 245–249.
—— (1981) Editorial. Cerebral laterality and psychopathology: fact and fiction. *Psychological Medicine*, **11**, 219–227.
GUSELLA, J. F., WEXLER, N. S., CONNEALLY, P. M., *et al* (1983) A polymorphic DNA marker genetically linked to Huntington's disease. *Nature*, **306**, 234–238.
GUR, R. E., GUR, R. C., SKOLNICK, B. E., *et al* (1985) Brain function in psychiatric disorders III. Regional cerebral blood flow in unmedicated schizophrenics. *Archives of General Psychiatry*, **42**, 329–334.
GUY, J. D., MAJORSKI, L. V., WALLACE, C. J., *et al* (1983) The incidence of minor physical anomalies in adult male schizophrenics. *Schizophrenia Bulletin*, **9**, 571–582.
HALL, L. D., LUCK, S. L., NORWOOD, T., *et al* (1986) Nuclear magnetic resonance spectroscopy–future technical prospects. In *New Brain Imaging Techniques and Psychopharmacology*, BAP monograph no. 9 (ed. M. R. Trimble). Oxford: Oxford University Press.
HARE, E. H. (1975a) Season of birth in schizophrenia and neurosis. *American Journal of Psychiatry*, **132**, 1168–1171.
—— (1975b) Manic depressive psychosis and season of birth. *Acta Psychiatrica Scandinavica*, **52**, 69–79.
—— & WALTER, S. D. (1978) Seasonal variation in admissions of psychiatric patients and its relation to seasonal variation in their births. *Journal of Epidemiology and Community Health*, **32**, 47–52.
HAUG, J. O. (1962) Pneumoencephalographic studies in mental disease. *Acta Psychiatrica Scandinavica* (suppl.), **165**, 381–114.
HAUSER, P., POLLOCK, B., FINKELBERG, F., *et al* (1985) On sinistrality and sex differences in schizophrenia. *American Journal of Psychiatry*, **142**, 1228.
HEINZ. R., MARTINE, Z. J. & HAENGGLI, A., (1977) Reversibility of cerebral atrophy in anorexia nervosa and Cushing's syndrome. *Journal of Computer Assisted Tomography*, **1**, 415–418.
HERTZIG, M. E. & BIRCH, H. G. (1966) Neurologic organisation in psychiatrically disturbed adolescent girls. *Archives of General Psychiatry*, **15**, 590–598.
—— & —— (1968) Neurologic organisation in psychiatrically disturbed adolescents. A comparative consideration of sex differences. *Archives of General Psychiatry*, **19**, 528–537.
HIMSWORTH, R. L., CARMEL, P. W. & FRANTZ, A. G. (1972) The location of the chemoreceptor controlling growth hormone secretion during hypoglycaemia in primates. *Endocrinology*, **91**, 217–226.
HODGKINSON, S., SHERRINGTON, R., GURLING, H., *et al* (1987) Molecular genetic evidence for heterogeneity in manic depression. *Nature*, **325**, 805–806.
HOLZMAN, P. S., PROCTOR, L. R. & HUGHES, D. W. (1973) Eye-tracking patterns in schizophrenia. *Science*, **181**, 179–181.
——, KRINGLEN, E., LEVY, D. L., *et al* (1977) Abnormal pursuit eye movements in schizophrenia: evidence for genetic marker. *Archives of General Psychiatry*, **34**, 802–805.
HORNYKIEWICZ, O. (1963) Topography and behaviour of noradrenaline and dopamine (3-hydroxytyramine) in the substantia nigra of normal and Parkinsonian patients. *Wiener Klinische Wochenschrift*, **75**, 309–312.

HOUNSFIELD, G. N. (1973) Computerised transverse axial scanning (tomography) part 1. Description of the system. *British Journal of Radiology*, **46**, 1106–1022.

JOHNSTONE, E. C. (1982) *Affective Disorders in Disorders of Neurohumoural Transmission* (ed. T. J. Crow) London: Academic Press.

——, CROW, T. J., FRITH, C. D., *et al* (1976) Cerebral ventricular size and cognitive impairment in chronic schizophrenia. *Lancet*, *ii*, 924–926.

——, BOURNE, R. C., CROW, T. J., *et al* (1981) The relationship between clinical response psychophysiological variables and plasma levels of amitriptyline and diazepam in enurotic out-patients. *Psychopharmacology*, **72**, 233–240.

—— & FERRIER, I. N. (1981) Neuroendocrine markers of CNS drug effects. In *Methods in Clinical Pharmacology–Central Nervous System* (eds M. H. Lader & A. Richens). London: Macmillan Press.

——, CROW, T. J., MACMILLAN, J. F., *et al* (1986a) A magnetic resonance study of early schizophrenia. *Journal of Neurology, Neurosurgery and Psychiatry*, **49**, 136–139.

——, OWENS, D. G. C., CROW, T. J., *et al* (1986b) Hypothyroidism as a correlate of lateral ventricular enlargement in manic depressive and neurotic illness. *British Journal of Psychiatry*, **148**, 317–321.

KOVELMAN, J. A. & SCHEIBEL, A. B. (1984) A neurohistological correlate of schizophrenia. *Biological Psychiatry*, **19**, 1601–1621.

KRAEPELIN, E. (1896) *Psychiatrie*, 5th edn. Leipzig: Barth.

KRETSCHMER, E. (1936) *Physique and Character–an Investigation of the Nature of Constitution and of the Theory of Temperament*. London: Kegan Paul, Trench, Trubner & Co. Ltd.

LADER, M. H., RON, M. & PETURSSON, H. (1984) Computed axial brain tomography in long term benzodiazepine users. *Psychological Medicine*, **14**, 203–206.

LAMBERT, T., CONNELLY, J., BJARNASON, I., *et al* (1987) Intestinal Permeability in Schizophrenia. Presented in Short Papers, Spring Quarterly Meeting of Royal College of Psychiatrists, Aberdeen.

LANCET (1978) The biochemistry of depression. *Lancet*, *i*, 422–423.

—— (1982) Adrenergic receptors in depression. *Lancet*, *i*, 781.

—— (1983) Gluten in schizophrenia. *Lancet*, *i*, 744–745.

—— (1984) Regional neuronal activity in schizophrenia. *Lancet*, *i*, 494.

LAPIN, I. P. & OXENKRUG, G. F. (1969) Intensification of the central serotoninergic processes as a possible determinant of the thymoleptic effect. *Lancet*, *i*, 132–136.

LISHMAN, W. A. & MCMEEKAN, E. R. L. (1976) Hand preference patterns in psychiatric patients. *British Journal of Psychiatry*, **129**, 158–166.

MCGUFFIN, P., FESTENSTEIN, H. & MURRAY, R. (1983) A family study of HLA antigens and other genetics markers in schizophrenia. *Psychological Medicine*, **13**, 31–43.

MCMANUS, I. C. (1981) Handedness and birth stress. *Psychological Medicine*, **11**, 485–496.

—— (1983) The interpretation of laterality. *Cortex*, **19**, 187–214.

—— (1984) Genetics of handedness in relation to language disorder. *Advances in Neurology*, **42**, 125–138.

MORIHISA, J. M., DUFFY, F. H. & WYATT, R. J. (1983) Brain electrical activity mapping (BEAM) in schizophrenic patients. *Archives of General Psychiatry*, **40**, 719–728.

MURPHY, D. L. & WYATT, R. J. (1972) Reduced monoamine oxidase activity in blood platelets from schizophrenic patients. *Nature*, **238**, 225–226.

NAGUIB, M., MCGUFFIN, P., LEVY, R., *et al* (1987) Genetic markers in late paraphrenia: a study of HLA antigens. *British Journal of Psychiatry*, **150**, 124–127.

NASRALLAH, H. A., KELLOR, K., VAN SCHROEDER, C., *et al* (1981) Motoric laterization in schizophrenic males. *American Journal of Psychiatry*, **138**, 114–1115.

NERL, C., MAYEUX, R. & O'NEILL, J. (1984) HLA-linked complement markers in Alzheimer's and Parkinson's disease: C4 variant (C4B2) a possible marker for senile dementia of the Alzheimer type. *Neurology (Cleveland)*, **34**, 310–314.

NOEL, G. L., SUK, H. K., STONE, G. J., *et al* (1972) Human prolactin and growth hormone release during surgery and other conditions of stress. *Journal of Clinical Endocrinology and Metabolism*, **35**, 840–851.

OBRIST, W. D., THOMSON, H. K., WANG, H. S., *et al* (1975) Regional cerebral blood flow estimated by [33]Xenon inhalation. *Stroke*, **6**, 245–256.

ODEGARD, O. (1974) Season of birth in the general population and in patients with mental disorder in Norway. *British Journal of Psychiatry*, **125**, 397–405.

64   *Research methods in psychiatry*

ORWIN, A., WRIGHT, C. E., HARDING, G. F. A., *et al* (1986) Serial visual evoked potential recordings in Alzheimer's disease. *British Medical Journal*, **293**, 9–10.

OSBORNE, M., CRAYTON, J. W., JAVAID, J., *et al* (1982) Lack of effect of a gluten-free diet on neuroleptic blood levels in schizophrenic patients. *Biological Psychiatry*, **17**, 627–629.

OWEN, F., CROSS, A. J., CROW, T. J., *et al* (1978) Increased dopamine receptor sensitivity in schizophrenia. *Lancet*, ii, 223–226.

——, BOURNE, R. C., CROW, T. J., *et al* (1981) Platelet monoamine oxidase activity in acute schizophrenia: relationship to symptomatology and neuroleptic medication. *British Journal of Psychiatry*, **139**, 16–22.

——, CRAWLEY, J., CROSS, A. J., *et al* (1985) Dopamine D$_2$ receptors and schizophrenia. In *Psychopharmacology: Recent Advances and Future Prospects* (ed. S. D. Iversen). Oxford: Oxford University Press.

OWENS, D. G. C. & JOHNSTONE, E. C. (1980) The disabilities of chronic schizophrenia–their nature and the factors contributing to their development. *British Journal of Psychiatry*, **136**, 384–395.

——, ——, CROW, T. J., *et al* (1985) Lateral ventricular size in schizophrenia: relationship to the disease process and its clinical manifestations. *Psychological Medicine*, **15**, 27–41.

PARE, C. M. B., YOUNG, D. P. H., PRICE, K., *et al* (1969) 5-hydroxytryptamine, noradrenaline and dopamine in brain stem hypothalamus and caudate nucleus of controls and patients committing suicide by coal gas poisoning. *Lancet*, ii, 133–135.

PECK, R. E. (1959) The SHP test–an aid in the detection and measurement of depression. *Archives of General Psychiatry*, **1**, 35–40.

QUITKIN, F., RIFKIN, A. & KLEIN, D. F. (1976). Neurological soft signs in schizophrenia and character disorders. Organicity in schizophrenia with premorbid associality and emotionally unstable character disorders. *Archives of General Psychiatry*, **33**, 845–853.

RENVOIZE, E. B. (1984) An HLA and family study of Alzheimer's disease. *Psychological Medicine*, **14**, 515–520.

RIEDER, R. O., MANN, L. S., WEINBERGER, D. R., *et al* (1983) Computed tomographic scans in patients with schizophrenia, schizo-affective and bipolar affective disorder. *Archives of General Psychiatry*, **40**, 735–739.

ROBERTS, G. W., POLAK, J. M. & CROW, T. J. (1984) Peptide circuitary of limbic system. In *Psychopharmacology of the Limbic System* (eds M. R. Trimble & E. Zarifian). Oxford: Oxford University Press.

ROBINSON, R. G., LIPSEY, J. R., BOLLA-WILSON, K., *et al* (1985) Mood disorders in left handed stroke patients. *American Journal of Psychiatry*, **142**, 1424–1429.

ROCHFORD, J. M., DETRE, T., TUCKER, G. J., *et al* (1970) Neuropsychological impairments in functional psychiatric diseases. *Archives of General Psychiatry*, **22**, 114–119.

ROSENBERG, J. B. & WELLER, G. M. (1973) Minor physical anomalies and academic performance in young school-children. *Developmental Medicine and Child Neurology*, **15**, 131–135.

RUBIN, R. T. (1977) Strategies of neuroendocrine research in psychiatry. In *Neuroregulators and Psychic Disorders* (eds E. Usdin, D. A. Harnsburg & J. D. Barches), pp. 233–241. New York: Oxford University Press.

SCHILDKRAUT, J. J. (1965) The catecholamine hypothesis–a review of the supporting evidence. *American Journal of Psychiatry*, **122**, 509–522.

SHAW, D. M., CAMPS, F. E. & ECCLESTON, D. G. (1967) 5-hydroxytryptamine in the hind brain of depressive suicides. *British Journal of Psychiatry*, **133**, 1407–1411.

SHEAR, K. M., KLIGFIELD, P., HARSHFIELD, G., *et al* (1987) Cardiac rate and rhythm in panic patients. *American Journal of Psychiatry*, **114**, 633–637.

SHELDON, W. H. (1942) *The Varieties of Temperament. A Psychology of Constitutional Differences.* New York: Harper and Brothers.

SHIMIZU, A., ENDO, M., TORII, H., *et al* (1985) Hand preference in schizophrenics and handedness conversion in their childhood. *Acta Psychiatrica Scandinavica*, **72**, 259–265.

SINGH, M. M. & KAY, S. R. (1976) Wheat gluten as a pathogenic factor in schizophrenia. *Science*, **191**, 401–402.

SNYDER, S. H., BANERJEE, S. P., YAMAMURA, A. I., *et al* (1974) Drugs, neurotransmitters and schizophrenia. *Science*, **184**, 1243–1253.

SOLOMON, C. M., HOLZMAN, P. S., LEVIN, S., *et al* (1987) The association between eye tracking dysfunctions and thought disorder in psychosis. *Archives of General Psychiatry*, **44**, 31–35.

STEINER, R. E. & BYDDER, G. M. (1984) Clinical nuclear magnetic resonance imaging. In *Recent Advances in Medicine*, no. 19 (eds A. M. Dawson, N. D. Compston & G. M. Besser). London: Churchill Livingstone.

STEVENS, J. R. (1982) Neuropathology of schizophrenia. *Archives of General Psychiatry*, **39**, 1131–1139.

ST GEORGE-HYSLOP, P. H., TANZI, R. E., POLINSKY, R. J., *et al* (1987) The genetic defect causing familial Alzheimer's disease maps on chromosome 21. *Science*, **235**, 885–890.

STOREY, P. (1966) Lumbar air encephalography in chronic schizophrenia: a controlled experiment. *British Journal of Psychiatry*, **122**, 135–144.

STRAIN, G. W. & STRAIN, J. J. (1978) Editorial. *Psychosomatic Medicine*, **40**, 2–4.

TAYLOR, P. J., DALTON, R. & FLEMINGER, J. J. (1980) Handedness in schizophrenia. *British Journal of Psychiatry*, **136**, 375–383.

——, ——, ——, *et al* (1982) Differences between two studies of hand preference in psychiatric patients. *British Journal of Psychiatry*, **140**, 166–173.

TAYLOR, C. B., SHEIKH, J., AGRAS, W. S., *et al* (1986) Ambulatory heart rate changes in patients with panic attacks. *American Journal of Psychiatry*, **143**, 478–482.

THASE, M. E., REYNOLDS, C. F., GLANZ, L. M., *et al* (1987) Nocturnal penile tumescence in depressed men. *American Journal of Psychiatry*, **144**, 89–92.

TYRER, P. & MACKAY, A., (1986) Schizophrenia: no longer a functional psychosis. *Trends in Neurosciences*, **9**, 537–538.

WALDROP, M. F., PEDERSON, F. A. & BELL, R. Q. (1968) Minor physical anomalies and behaviour in preschool children. *Child Development*, **39**, 391–400.

WALKER, H. A. (1977) Incidence of minor physical anomaly in autism. *Journal of Autism and Childhood Schizophrenia*, **7**, 165–176.

WEINBERGER, D. R., WAGNER, R. L. & WYATT, R. J. (1983) Neuropathological studies of schizophrenia a selective review. *Schizophrenia Bulletin*, **9**, 193–212.

WOOD, K. & COPPEN, A. (1985) Platelet transport and receptor sites in depressive illness. In *Psychopharmacology: Recent Advances and Future Prospects* (ed. S. D. Iversen). Oxford: Oxford University Press.

WOOD, N. C., HAMILTON, I., AXON, A. T. R., *et al* (1987) Abnormal intestinal permeability: an aetiological factor in chronic psychiatric disorders? *British Journal of Psychiatry*, **150**, 853–856.

YANNITSI, S., LIAKOS, A. & PAPAKOSTAS, Y. (1987) Electrodermal responding and chlorpromazine treatment in schizophrenia. *British Journal of Psychiatry*, **150**, 850–853.

YEN, S. C. (1977) Neuroendocrine aspects of the regulation of cyclic gonadotroplin release in women. In *Clinical Neuroendocrinology* (eds L. Martin & G. M. Besser), pp. 175–196. New York: Academic Press.

YOUNG, I. R., HALL, A. S., PALLIS, C. A., *et al* (1981) Nuclear magnetic resonance imaging of the brain in multiply sclerosis. *Lancet*, **ii**, 1063–1066.

ZARCONE, V. P., BENSON, K. L. & BERGER, P. A. (1987) Abnormal rapid eye movement latencies in schizophrenia. Archives of General Psychiatry, **44**, 45–48.

Further reading

Papers

EGELAND, J. A. & HOSTETTER, A. M. (1983) Amish study, I: Affective disorders among the Amish 1979–1980. *American Journal of Psychiatry*, **140**, 56–61.

——, —— & ESHLEMAN, S. K. (1983) Amish study, III: The impact of cultural factors on diagnosis of bipolar illness. *American Journal of Psychiatry*, **140**, 67–71.

HOSTETTER, A. M., EGELAND, J. A. & ENDICOTT, J. (1983) Amish study, II: Consensus diagnoses and reliability results. *American Journal of Psychiatry*, **140**, 62–66.

KAY, D. W. K. (1986) The genetics of Alzheimer's disease. *British Medical Bulletin*, **42**, 19–23.

KETY, S. S. (1959) Biochemical theories of schizophrenia. *Science*, **129**, 1528–1532.

McGUFFIN, P. (1980) What have transplant antigens got to do with psychosis? *British Journal of Psychiatry*, **136**, 511–512.

WATT, D. C. (1982) The search for genetic linkage in schizophrenia. *British Journal of Psychiatry*, **140**, 532–537.

Books

FLOR-HENRY, P. & GRUZELIER, J. H. (eds) (1983) *Laterality and Psychopathology. Developments in Psychiatry*, vol. 6. Amsterdam: Elsevier Science Publishers.

IVERSEN, S. D. (ed.) (1985) *Psychopharmacology: Recent Advances and Future Prospects*, BAP monograph no. 6. Oxford: Oxford University Press.

LADER, M. (ed.) (1975) *The Psychophysiology of Mental Illness*. London: Routledge and Kegan Paul.

TRIMBLE, M. R. (ed.) (1986) *New Brain Imaging Techniques and Psychopharmacology*, BAP monograph no. 9. Oxford: Oxford University Press.

4 Epidemiological methods in psychiatry

SIMON BACKETT and ANDREW ROBINSON

The aim of this chapter is to examine some of the basic principles of epidemiology, and to consider how these may be applied in psychiatric research. The primary concern is with epidemiological methods and concepts, and no attempt is made to review the epidemiology of specific psychiatric illnesses.

The term 'epidemiology' can be used in either a broad or narrow sense; the narrow is the more scientific and familiar, while the broad use tends to be more interesting but at the same time may be misleading. Psychiatric epidemiology can be defined as "the branch of psychiatric research that investigates how mental illness is distributed in the population, and the factors that influence that distribution". Other definitions of epidemiology, for instance that it is "the numerate branch of human ecology" or "the study of the mass aspects of disease", suggest a broader area of interest and each draws attention to certain important features of the research approach. The first and perhaps most important of these features is the distinction between epidemiological and clinical studies. Clinical studies are chiefly involved in describing illness affecting individual patients, while epidemiological studies stand back from the individual and consider the illness or event in relation to the population in which it occurs. This primary interest in the population as opposed to the individual means that the epidemiologist is concerned with all members in the group, irrespective of whether or not they are ill or have come to medical attention.

A second important feature of the approach is that the method is essentially comparative, so that a problem is examined by comparing the frequency of particular phenomena or illnesses in different groups in the population. One of the primary tasks of the psychiatric epidemiologist is to search for the aetiology or causes of mental illness, and this is achieved by identifying features of the physical or social environment that are associated with the illness under investigation. Once identified, that association is examined in greater detail, a process which is aimed at revealing its nature and more importantly whether the relationship is causal or non-causal. Finally it should be emphasised that the epidemiological method is always numerical. Since descriptions are stated quantitatively and because associations are demonstrated statistically, statistical methods are an essential component of an epidemiological approach.

The application of epidemiological methods

Knowledge of the distribution of an illness or event in a population can be used to increase our understanding of the causes of disease and how they can be most effectively managed. It should be emphasised that a single method of investigation may serve more than one objective.

The search for causal factors

A principal concern of epidemiological research has been to investigate the factors that cause illness. An awareness of the determinants of a disease is important for two reasons. In the first instance the information contributes to an understanding of the overall clinical picture; secondly, and perhaps more importantly, it may help to indicate the way that illness can be prevented. Because prevention of illness is one of the basic concerns of epidemiology, particular interest is centred on those determinants of the disease that can be manipulated or altered in some way. This is in contrast to other determinants, for instance the genetic constitution, which are less amenable to change, and, although of general interest, cannot easily be incorporated in a preventive strategy.

The investigation of the natural history of an illness

Goldberg & Huxley (1980) in *The Pathway to Psychiatric Care* have described some of the factors that influence the extent, timing and outcome of the doctor/patient contact. Because this contact is both variable and intermittent the picture obtained by the doctor is often incomplete. A full understanding of the natural history of an illness, with particular attention to the eventual outcome, is essential information if the doctor is to recommend appropriate treatment. For instance a considerable amount is known about the short-term outcome of many of the major psychiatric illnesses. Much less is known about what effects these illnesses have on the individual in the long term.

Example: depression

A recent study by Lee & Murray (1988) looked at the long-term outcome of a group of patients with a primary depressive illness. Each of these patients had been involved in an earlier study by Kendell (1968), who had examined the outcome and had concluded that those patients with psychotic features tended to respond better to biological treatments, with the result that they had a comparatively good short-term outcome. When the patients were reassessed 18 years later, a number of important changes had taken place. Fewer than one-fifth of the survivors had remained well in the intervening years and over a third of the series had either committed suicide or had experienced chronic distress and handicap. Those with a psychotic illness were more likely to have been readmitted to hospital and the overall prognosis of this group, which had previously been thought to be comparatively good, now appeared very much worse than their neurotic counterparts.

It is this kind of information, in which the clinical picture is completed and in which the natural history of the illness is fully understood, that is essential for the doctor to be aware of if he/she is to make a rational decision about which form of therapy to recommend.

The classification of illness

The epidemiological characteristics of an illness, which include a description of the distribution of factors such as age, gender, social class and ethnic background, are part of the basic description of diseases and can be used to help distinguish one condition from another. For example, an examination of the extensive literature on anorexia nervosa shows that much of it is based on the descriptions of small series of patients and that many of these cases have been selected because of some feature of special interest. While this information is undoubtedly important and contributes to our understanding of the scope and boundaries of the symptoms involved, it is impossible to say whether the features described are unique to the individual or are representative of all cases. To examine the possible aetiological factors that contribute to anorexia nervosa it is essential to know how common the symptoms of a representative sample of cases are and about their distribution in the population.

Example: anorexia nervosa (Kendell et al, 1973)

Early reports on anorexia nervosa suggested that the condition was to be found most commonly among young middle-class women, occurred rarely in negroes, and that the incidence was increasing. These findings had important implications from both an aetiological and health care planning point of view, and in an attempt to establish the validity of these clinical impressions Kendell *et al* studied a large sample of patients with this diagnostic label. The patients were selected from psychiatric registers in three geographical areas: the north-east of Scotland, the Camberwell district in London and Monro County in New York State. The results provided the first basic epidemiological data on anorexia nervosa and as such contributed considerably to our current knowledge of the condition and the associated symptoms. The study demonstrated a disparity in the figures from two of the centres, which raised the question as to whether these were real differences in the incidence rate or whether these differences were the result of varying diagnostic criteria. Although this issue remained, they concluded that there did appear to be a condition with a recognisable constellation of symptoms and that the incidence was similar in the three areas.

Testing the efficacy and efficiency of health care intervention at both a preventive and a curative level

All treatments or methods of intervention need to be examined and epidemiological methods can contribute to this evaluation. The efficacy of health care intervention involves an estimation of the extent to which a specific therapy or preventive strategy produces a beneficial result. Efficacy is a measure of the effectiveness of an intervention, such as a new drug or treatment programme, which as a result can be compared with other forms of intervention with similar aims. In contrast the efficiency is a measure of the effort expended in terms of money, resources and time to carry out an intervention of known efficacy. The ability to measure each of these elements is of crucial importance in health provision.

Assistance in health care prediction and planning by determining the frequency and distribution of disorders

Knowledge of the aetiology, natural history, frequency and distribution of various illnesses is essential for the health care planner who is faced with the task of matching need with available resources.

Case definition

One of the fundamental tasks for the epidemiologist is to estimate the frequency, in other words the incidence or prevalence, of illness in populations and to test for differences between the rates for defined subgroups. Although this may at first appear to be a straightforward exercise it raises the question of "what is a case?" or "how is the illness defined?". The problems associated with case definition concern both clinicians and research workers and involve all areas of medicine, since it is now recognised that disease in populations tends to exist as a continuum of severity rather than as discrete phenomena (Rose & Barker, 1979). This issue, although relevant to medical research in general, has posed a particular problem for psychiatry and for psychiatric epidemiology. For instance, when psychiatrists use labels such as 'anxiety' or 'depression', are they describing the same clinical phenomenon and, furthermore, is there agreement on what symptoms are required before such an illness can be diagnosed? These are important questions for the epidemiologist because there must be uniformity in these definitions if meaningful conclusions are to be drawn by comparing rates between populations. Similarly, if the relationships between illness and certain social or environmental factors of possible aetiological importance are to be investigated, then again it is essential that there is agreement about what constitutes a case.

Considerable progress has been made over the past 15 years, with the development of standardised psychiatric interview schedules and psychiatric screening questionnaires, which have allowed researchers to examine systematically the distribution of symptoms in patients. The principal psychiatric interview schedule in use in the UK is the Present State Examination (PSE) developed by Wing *et al* (1974). The interview inquires into the presence of a number of psychiatric symptoms and when this information is incorporated into a computer program known as CATEGO (Wing & Sturt, 1978) it will give a CATEGO class and a psychiatric (ICD-9) diagnosis. A more recent development has been the Index of Definition (ID), which is a measure of the certainty with which a psychiatric diagnosis can be made based on the information gathered in the PSE interview. There are eight levels to this scale, ranging from no symptoms (ID1), to threshold 'caseness' (ID5), to definite 'caseness' (ID6-8). Those with an ID of 5 or greater are considered to be psychiatrically ill and can be assigned both a CATEGO class and an ICD diagnosis.

In the United States similar structured interviews have been designed. The first to be based on operational definitions were developed in St Louis and were known as the Feighner criteria (Feighner *et al*, 1972). These criteria were subsequently elaborated by Spitzer *et al* (1978) to produce the Research Diagnostic Criteria, which themselves have formed the basis of a structured interview schedule designed to rate clinical features, known as the Schedule for Affective Disorders and Schizophrenia (SADS). An additional version, and SADS/L, has also been developed so that lifetime prevalence of diagnoses could be made for those subjects who were not in a current episode of illness. More elaborate and detailed interview schedules have been designed and continue to undergo evaluation, and as they develop are assessed for their suitability in a variety of settings and with different patient groups.

While it is essential that there is agreement on what constitutes a 'case', there is a parallel need for the reliable definition of social and environmental variables. Again there have been major advances in these areas, most notable among them being the measurement of life events. Using the Bedford College Life Events and Difficulties Schedule (LEDS), Brown & Harris (1978) have demonstrated the major aetiological role life events play in the onset of depressive illness.

Measures of psychiatric morbidity

In order to make comparisons between populations meaningful, the numbers of events or affected individuals are rarely considered on their own and are usually described in relation to the population from which they are drawn. This relationship is referred to as a 'rate' and is an estimate of the ratio between the number of persons or events (the numerator) and the total population at risk for that event (the denominator): the numerator contains the number of subjects experiencing a disease or some other event, while the denominator refers to the population from which the numerator is derived (the population at risk).

There are two kinds of rate and the distinction between them is important. In the first, the *true* rate, both numerator and denominator are derived from the same population. Table 4.1 shows the relationship between parasuicide rates and employment status. The denominators used to calculate these rates are taken from the mid-year population estimates for Edinburgh City, supplied by the General Register Office, Scotland. These are true rates because all subjects counted in the numerator appear also in the denominator. It is important to note that in this instance the denominator is not the total number of men, but the number of economically active men in the city within a specified age group, who are then the true population at risk. The second or 'false' rate refers to those situations in which the numerator and denominator originate from different populations. A frequently cited example is the admission rate to a hospital, in which the numerator is the number of admissions, which are events, not people, and the denominator is an estimate of the population from which those admissions originate. Illogical conclusions may be drawn if the two kinds of rate are confused and comparisons are made between them. It should also be emphasised that there are different types of numerator. The terms may refer to the total number of events or episodes, for example admissions to a hospital, where the same individual can be counted on more than one occasion. Alternatively there is the unduplicated count of the number of individuals experiencing that illness or event during a defined period. In this case the individuals in question are counted only once, regardless of how many episodes may have occurred. Each numerator will have its own unique characteristics and care must be taken when making comparisons to ensure that they are not confused (see Fig. 4.1).

TABLE 4.1
Parasuicide patient rates by employment status, 1982–85, per 100 000 economically active males (aged 16 and over) in Edinburgh City

	1982	1983	1984	1985
Employed	115	111	123	109
Unemployed	1344	1051	926	986

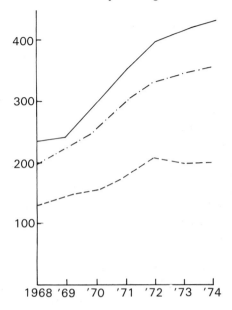

Fig. 4.1 Edinburgh male parasuicide rates (per 100 000 population per year): ———— , *no. of admissions;* —— · —— , *no. of patients;* — — — , *no. of first admissions (Holding et al, 1977)*

Prevalence and incidence rates

In epidemiological studies the two most commonly used measures of disease frequency are prevalence and incidence. The point prevalence rate refers to the proportion of people in a defined population who are affected by the disorder at a particular point in time. This involves a single or cross-sectional measurement of the number of affected individuals in a population and is expressed either as a percentage or a rate per 1000 at risk.

To illustrate this Fig. 4.2 represents ten individuals, each of whom has developed an illness at some point over a period of three years. The horizontal lines represent the duration of the illness of each individual. Assume there are a further 90 individuals in the population under examination who did not develop the illness. On a day at the end of year 1 it can be seen that five out of the population of 100 were affected and as a result the point prevalence rate was 5%. At the end of year 3 the point prevalence rate was 4%.

In an illness such as schizophrenia, in which the course is often one of a series of relapses and remissions, a single measurement such as the point prevalence rate would tend to underestimate the frequency of that condition, and a more appropriate measurement would be the period prevalence rate. This is defined as the proportion of people who are affected by a disorder at any time within a stated period. Thus the period prevalence rate for the

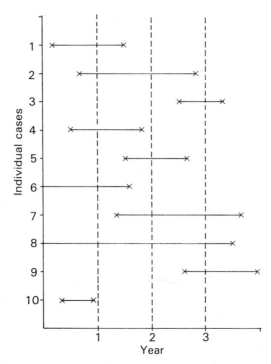

Fig. 4.2   Episodes of psychiatric illness in a hypothetical population (total population 100: 90 individuals did not become ill and do not appear in the figure)

year refers to the total number of individuals experiencing that illness at any time during that year. In Fig. 4.2 for year 2 the period prevalence rate is 7% and for year 3 is 6%.

The inception or incidence rate is a measure of new episodes of illness and is the proportion of formerly well subjects who develop an illness in a defined period of time (usually a year). Because the measures of incidence start with a group who are initially free of an illness and only counts those who subsequently become affected, the rate so derived gives valuable information about the future likelihood or risk of an illness developing. In Fig. 4.2 the incidence rate for year 1 is 4% and for year 2 is 2%.

Prevalence is often likened to the 'pool' of illness with new cases introduced into this pool by the incidence of that illness. Recovery, death and migration lead to the outflow so that a relationship exists between the incidence, prevalence and duration of an illness:

prevalence = incidence × duration of illness

For example, parasuicide is a behaviour that occurs in discrete episodes with, in most cases, the patient remaining in hospital only briefly. Under these circumstances the incidence and period prevalence are roughly the same. In contrast, more chronic conditions such as schizophrenia tend to have a low incidence but a comparatively high prevalence rate.

Ingham & Miller (1976) have proposed an alternative approach to the concept of prevalence that may have particular relevance to psychiatry. They described the problems of defining the boundaries of an illness and the often arbitrary decisions associated with placing a cut-off point, the nature of the severity continuum itself and the factors that influence psychiatric referral. As a result they argued that prevalence statements such as "*x*% of the general population is mentally ill" should be treated with caution. Instead, they suggested that a rate should be expressed in dimensional terms and that differing degrees of severity of a symptom, such as distress or depression, could be quantified and the distribution curves of these individual symptoms compared.

Sampling methods

Epidemiological studies are aimed at understanding the characteristics of a whole population. In most cases it is not possible to examine the entire group and it will be necessary to select one or more samples or subsets of that population. It may not matter that only a section of the population is being examined, and in fact it can be argued that it is preferable to obtain detailed information on a small number of subjects rather than poorer-quality data on a large number.

If it is the researcher's intention to extrapolate the findings from the sample to the whole population, then the sample must be as representative and unbiased as possible. These unbiased methods are collectively known as 'probability sampling', and the most frequently used are the simple random sample and the systematic sample. In each of these the selection process is similar to drawing lots, in that it ensures that each subject in the population has an equal chance of being selected for the sample.

It must be emphasised that a sample is only an approximation of the population from which it is derived and that however good the sampling procedure is, the properties of the sample will never be exactly the same as those of the population.

The simple random sample

A random sample is identified from a complete list of all members of the target population, otherwise known as a sampling frame. The amount that a random sample will differ from the 'true' population value is measured by the standard error. This is a property of the sample mean and is a measure of its accuracy as an estimate of the population mean.

Example (Priest, 1971)

A simple random sample was used in a study designed to examine the prevalence of psychiatric illness among the single homeless in Edinburgh. It was estimated that at the time there were about 900 homeless people living in or around the centre of the city. Using the three largest common-lodging houses, and numbering the beds in each house, a sample of 98 subjects was selected using random-number tables. To counter the argument that these three lodging houses were not representative of the total homeless population, the social and demographic data of the subjects selected for the study were compared with, and shown to be similar to, those given in a separate national survey of the homeless. From this it was concluded that they were representative, and that it was valid to make statements about the homeless population in general based on the information collected in this study.

The systematic sample

An easier method to undertake, and one that often provides adequate representativeness, is the systematic sample. With a random start, the sample is collected by selecting every nth number from the sampling frame, depending on the size of the sample required. In some situations the systematic sample has many practical advantages over the random sample and may be equally representative.

The stratified sample

Another example of probability sampling is the stratified sample. This method is used in situations in which, because of the distribution of variables within the population, the researcher requires a particular subgroup to be either over- or under-represented. The population is divided into strata, for instance age or sex groups, or diagnostic categories, and a random sample is selected from each of these strata.

Example (Dyer & Kreitman, 1984)

In a study designed to examine suicidal intent in a group of parasuicides it was considered important to examine the whole population – all age groups and both sexes. It is known that there is a preponderance of younger women among parasuicides which would be reflected in a random sample. In order to include a sufficient number of older men the sample was stratified by sex and age group and a random sample then selected from each stratum.

Multistage sampling

Finally, multistage sampling is a method that involves more than one stage of sampling, using some or all of the techniques described. If the distribution of a variable in a large geographical area is being examined, the first sample may involve the selection of units, such as electoral regions or other boundaries, within a city. Having established these initial units it becomes possible to list and sample more basic units, such as households or individuals. To give an example, to examine the prevalence of minor psychiatric morbidity in the setting of a general practice in a large city, at least two or possibly more stages would be required. Firstly, the sampling frame would be established by enumerating all the practices in the city and then using either a random or systematic method, a sample of practices would be identified. The second stage would involve selecting individuals from this sample, which could be achieved by using the sample practices' age/sex registers. In this example it should be remembered that practices often serve well defined geographical areas, which may themselves be associated with distinct social characteristics, and careful consideration would need to be given to the first-stage sampling to ensure that the practices selected were representative of the whole population.

Non-random sampling

There are certain situations in which probability sampling is impractical and a non-probability or non-random method may be used. The investigation of the misuse of illegal drugs provides an example since it poses particular problems for the researcher in the identification of the target population. Conventional surveys of self-reported drug use give some insight into the problem but are often dependent on the individual being willing to volunteer information. Since many may not be prepared to make this contribution, certain important sections of the drug-user population may be missed. In this situation a non-random method of contact known as 'snowballing' has been used and this has been able to provide valuable information, since it circumvents many of the constraints imposed by conventional surveys (Morrison, 1988). The method involves the researchers making contact with one or more people in the group in whose behaviour they are interested. By establishing a relationship of trust with certain 'key' individuals, the researchers will be guided and introduced to other members of the relevant social group until a large enough sample has been contacted. The success of the method is very much dependent upon the personal characteristics of the researchers and their ability to establish an appropriate and trusting relationship.

Sample size

When a study is being planned it is often the case that attention is centred on the practical issues associated with the collection of data and too little consideration is given to the likely results or the statistical analyses that will be required. This is an important area that must be addressed at the design stage otherwise there is a danger that either too many, or more likely too few, patients or events will be measured. If the sample is too small it will become apparent only when the study has been completed that there are insufficient data to support or refute the original hypotheses. To calculate the required sample size it will be necessary to be aware of the frequency of the event to be examined, and the accuracy to which it is to be measured. If there is any doubt in the mind of the researcher on this issue it is wise to seek statistical advice at an early stage in the planning process (see Chapter 2).

Measures of risk

Risk is a term usually associated with estimating the probability of some hazardous or unfavourable situation. It is a concept in epidemiology for estimating the likelihood of an outcome, for instance the probability of becoming ill or dying within a stated period of time or by a certain age. Risk factors have been defined in three ways: firstly as risk markers, that is, as an attribute that is associated with a specified outcome but not necessarily as a causal factor; secondly as a determinant of an outcome, that is, where a causal relationship is proposed between factor and outcome; and thirdly, as a determinant modified by an intervention that reduces the risk of an outcome. Thus it is helpful always to include a definition of the way in which it is being used.

The value of measuring risk lies in the estimation of the relative importance of a risk factor and the aetiology or outcome of a disease. High-risk groups may be identified, and thus resources can be deployed efficiently. Relative risk and odds ratios are used to measure the strength of an association between a risk factor and a disease. Measures that take into account not only the strength of effect of exposure but also the number exposed to the risk factor are commonly termed 'attributable risk' (see Waltner-Toews (1982) for other names and operational definitions).

Relative risk

The relative or excess risk is the ratio of the incidence of an outcome in those who are exposed to a certain risk factor compared with the incidence in an unexposed group. In other words, it is a measure of how much more prone those who have been exposed to a risk factor are to have a given effect, compared with those who have not been exposed.

Calculation of the relative risk

$$\text{Relative risk} = \frac{\text{incidence in the exposed}}{\text{incidence in the unexposed}}$$

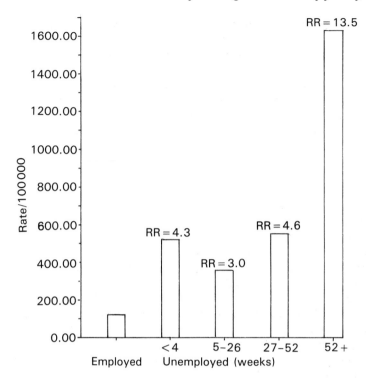

Fig. 4.3 Parasuicide rates by duration of unemployment, for Edinburgh City males, 1984 (RR = relative risk)

Figure 4.3 shows the parasuicide rates for employed and unemployed economically active males aged 16–65 years in Edinburgh during 1984 who were admitted to hospital following parasuicide. The relative risk of parasuicide for the long-term unemployed (more than 52 weeks) is about three times that for those cohorts who have been unemployed for less than one year and 14 times the rate for the employed. The different categories of unemployment are risk markers for parasuicide.

For cohort studies, relative risk is calculated as:

$$\text{relative risk (cohort studies)} = [a/(a+b)]/[c/(c+d)]$$
$$= a(c+d)/c(a+b)$$

Exposed	*Case*	*Non-case*	*Total*
Yes	a	b	$a+b$
No	c	d	$c+d$
Total	$a+c$	$b+d$	

Similarly, exit life events have been found to be risk markers for parasuicides and depression in the six months following that event (Paykel, 1980) (see Table 4.2).

TABLE 4.2
The relative risks of parasuicide, depression or schizophrenia in the six months following an exit event

Exits in last six months	
Suicide attempts	6.7
Depression	6.5
Schizophrenia	3.9
All events in last six months	
Suicide attempts	6.3
Depression	5.4
Schizophrenia	3.0
All events in last month	
Suicide attempts	10.0

Relative risk approximation for case-control studies is calculated as:

$$\text{relative risk (case control)} = \frac{a/(a + c)}{c/(a + c)} \div \frac{b(b + d)}{d(b + d)} = \frac{a/c}{b/d}$$

Odds ratio

Odds ratio (relative odds) is akin to relative risk, being the ratio of the odds of disease in exposed individuals relative to the unexposed:

$$\text{odds ratio } (a/c)/(b/d) = a \times d/b \times c$$

Odds ratio is used generally for rare diseases or outcomes, as it is simpler to apply and more closely approximates to the relative risk. Secondly, it can be used for either cohort studies or case-control studies. A fuller explanation is given by Schlesselman (1982).

Attributable risk

The attributable risk is the proportion of the disease in an exposed population that can be attributed to that exposure (McMahon & Pugh, 1970). It is the additional risk that follows exposure to the risk factor in excess of that experienced by the unexposed and is derived by subtracting the incidence of the disease among the unexposed from the corresponding rate among the exposed. Attributable risk can be used to estimate the proportional reduction of a disease in a population if exposure to the risk factor were prevented (Walter, 1978).

Population attributable risk per cent

While both the relative risk and attributable risk are useful measures of association, from a clinical point of view the population attributable risk per cent (PAR%) is perhaps the easiest to understand. It can be defined as the maximum percentage of an outcome in a population, that can be attributed directly to exposure to the risk factor.

TABLE 4.3

Parasuicide rates among employed and unemployed males, and measures of population attributable risk and risk percent, Edinburgh City

	Parasuicide rate per 100 000			
Year	Among all economically active (a)	Among employed (b)	Population attributable risk (a − b)	PAR% (a − b/a) × 100%
1968	172	98	74	43.2
1972	252	141	111	44.0
1976	299	173	126	42.0
1980	260	143	117	45.0
1984	247	123	124	50.2
1986	237	100	137	57.8

Table 4.3 gives the population attributable risk and risk percent arising out of unemployment for males in Edinburgh City for some years in the period 1968–86. Using 1986 as a worked example to illustrate this, we find 307 parasuicides among the economically active, of whom 199 were unemployed. The mid-year estimate of the economically active population of the city was 129 279 and the estimated employed population was 107 784. The rate of parasuicides per 100 000 among all the economically active was 237 and among the employed was 100. The population attributable risk was 237 − 100 = 137 and the PAR% was 137/237 × 100 = 57.8.

The figures illustrate that unemployment is a risk factor of increasing importance in parasuicide in Edinburgh since 1968 but cannot in itself be assumed to be a unitary cause as its effects are likely to be mediated through associated risk factors such as poverty or pessimism.

Standardisation

Comparing or contrasting rates between areas or over time may be misleading unless some account is taken of likely confounding factors. For example, age, sex and social class may have an association with depression and certainly have an association with parasuicidal behaviour; thus the age, sex and social-class structures of respective populations would have to be taken into account when comparing rates. Cross-tabulation is the simplest adjustment and will yield specific rates but can be cumbersome. Adjusted or standardised rates are used, therefore, to yield a summary rate. Two methods commonly used are direct and indirect standardisation.

Direct standardisation

Direct standardisation employs a weighted average of the specific rates in each period. The weights are equal to the proportion of the population in

TABLE 4.4
Direct standardisation of male suicide rates for Scotland, 1975

Age: years	Male suicides (deaths/100 000) (a)	% of reference population in age group (b)	a × b
15–19	2.78	11.7	32.53
20–24	11.34	10.0	113.40
25–34	9.75	18.3	178.42
35–44	12.76	15.7	200.33
45–54	15.72	16.2	254.66
55–64	16.35	13.9	227.26
65 +	14.51	14.2	206.04
		100	1212.64/100 = 12.13

each category in a convenient reference population. This is illustrated with reference to male suicide rates for Scotland in 1975 (Table 4.4).

Trends across time can be followed using these summary rates based on the initial year. This is illustrated by patient parasuicide rates for women

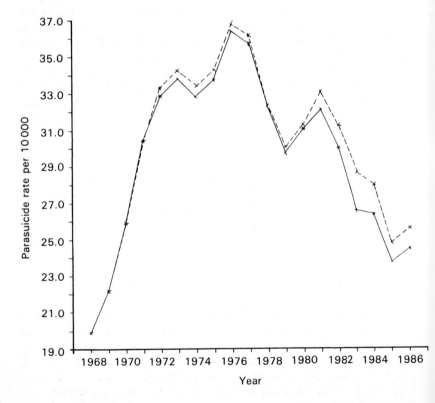

Fig. 4.4   Female patient parasuicide rates (per 10 000) 1968–86 admitted to the RPTC, Edinburgh (——, standardised; --- crude rate)

aged over 15 admitted to the Regional Poisoning Treatment Centre (RPTC) in Edinburgh from 1968 to 1986 (Fig. 4.4). In general, with such data sets, divergence of crude and standardised rates is apparent only after quite a lapse of time.

Indirect standardisation

The direct method of standardisation needed data on the constituent groups, the illustration of the number of suicides per age group and the breakdown of the reference population by age group. When that information is not available or where the rates are subject to large fluctuations, for example because an event is rare, the method of indirect standardisation can be applied.

A suitable reference population is chosen in which the rates for each group are known. Pooled data from all centres in a study could be used, for example. To illustrate this, a family doctor tests his impression that parasuicide is significantly commoner than expected in his group practice. He assumes that social class, age and sex are important but finds only the first to be so. The worked example for social class follows (see Table 4.5). He finds 12 parasuicides in his group practice over a year, thus the relative risk or standardised prevalence ratio adjusted for social class is 12/8 = 150%. He has no social class I + II parasuicides but has nine social class IV + V parasuicides. The ratio for classes IV + V is 9/5.3 = 170%. He concludes that his social class IV + V patients have an excess loading for parasuicide and might then consider other risk factors, such as long-term unemployment.

TABLE 4.5
Worked example of indirect standardisation by social class for parasuicide in a general practice

Social class	Number of patients in the practice	Yearly prevalence in reference population	Expected cases
I + II	1500	0.02%	0.3
III M + NM	3000	0.08%	2.4
IV	2000	0.13%	2.6
V	1000	0.27%	2.7
Total			8.0

Another summary statistic used frequently by the Registrar General and often by health boards is the standardised mortality ratio (SMR). The mortality rate for all classes is taken as a standard and this is applied to the mortality of a particular group. The ratio of the number of deaths observed in the study population is compared with the number of deaths expected if it had the same structure as the standard population. The observed deaths are then expressed as a percentage of the 'expected' deaths. Table 4.6 shows the SMRs by liver cirrhosis for different occupations.

TABLE 4.6
SMRs for liver cirrhosis among British males by occupation (1979–80, 1982–83)[1]

Occupational group	Standardised mortality rate
Average occupation	100
Publicans	1017
Deck, engine-room hands, bargemen, lightermen, boatmen	873
Barmen	612
Deck, engineering and radio officers and pilots, ship	417
Electrical engineers (so described)	387
Hotel and residential club managers	342
Innkeepers	315
Fishermen	296
Chefs, cooks	265
Restaurateurs	263
Authors, writers, journalists	261
Drivers, mates	225
Winders, reelers	202
Other domestic and school helpers	141
Garage proprietors	140
Medical practitioners	115
Farm workers	45
Printing machine minders and assistants	32
Managers in building and contracting	22

Source: Office of Population Censuses and Surveys (1986) and taken from Plant (1987).
1. Data aggregated for the two periods.

Investigative strategies

The methods of study in epidemiology follow certain strategies and may be categorised in a number of ways. Firstly they can be divided into either *observational* or *intervention* studies. Observational studies or surveys examine events in populations that occur naturally, while experimental or intervention studies consider a situation that has been deliberately arranged or manipulated. An observational approach might be used to demonstrate the presence of abnormal or involuntary movements and their association with neuroleptic medication, and following this an experimental study could then allocate the patients to different treatment groups to evaluate which form of therapy is most effective. As a general rule, observational studies are able to demonstrate where potentially important associations may lie and suggest directions for further research, while experimental studies provide more conclusive evidence of the nature of the relationship. It is the evidence presented by experimental studies that is usually required before changes take place in clinical practice.

Epidemiological studies may also be categorised as either *descriptive* or *analytical*. A descriptive study describes the patterns of disease distribution in a population and is able to determine the frequency of that illness, who experiences it, and where and when it occurs. Factors influencing the occurrence of a disease may be hypothesised, although causation can rarely

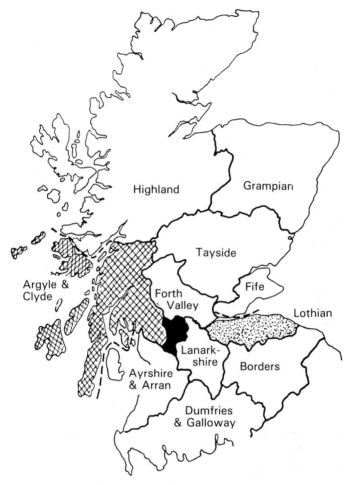

Fig. 4.5   Alcohol-related liver cirrhosis deaths for 1979–84: age-standardised ratios, for males aged over 25. □ *, ratio < 1.0;* ▨ *, ratio 1.0–1.25;* ▩ *, ratio 1.25–1.5;* ■ *, ratio > 1.5 (Greater Glasgow)*

be demonstrated. For example, certain geographical areas within Scotland have been observed to have significant differences in the mortality rate following cirrhosis of the liver and these have led to suggestions that there may be distinct regional patterns in drinking habits, diet, or even hepatitis B infection (Kreitman & Duffy, 1989).

In contrast, analytical studies are planned investigations designed to test specific hypotheses about the factors that influence an illness, for instance why one person is affected by an illness while another is not. In an analytical study the individuals may be classified in relation to the presence or absence of a specific disease or according to factors such as age, sex and marital status.

The aim of an analytical study is to define causes or determinants of disease more precisely than is possible by the descriptive method.

Finally, epidemiological studies may be described as either *retrospective* or *prospective*. In retrospective studies the researcher examines past events or experiences, collecting data from sources such as case notes, hospital admission records, or by interview. Prospective studies involve the identification and follow-up of a population and are often involved in examining the factors that influence the outcome of an illness. There are a number of methodological problems associated with each of these approaches. Prospective studies have the advantage of being able to collect relatively unbiased data, although it should be emphasised that bias may occur in the assessment of outcome. Set against this is the limitation that if the condition or event under examination is rare, a large number of subjects may need to be studied and a considerable lapse in time required for significant differences between the cohorts to become apparent. Each of these factors is likely to add considerably to the cost of the total project. In addition, subjects may be lost in the follow-up period, a fact that may itself distort the population, since those subjects who drop out of studies are often unrepresentative of the group as a whole. In contrast, retrospective studies, although usually less expensive, may suffer from incomplete recording of data or biased recall among subjects being interviewed. These issues are important and inevitably impose limitations on the ability to compare the results of both retrospective and prospective studies.

There are four main strategies commonly used in epidemiological research, and these are discussed under separate headings, below.

Cross-sectional studies

Cross-sectional studies are observational and descriptive, and are used to measure the prevalence of an illness or event. The essential element of a cross-sectional study is that only a single measurement is made. The consequence of this is that while the information gathered is able to provide a relatively quick and economical examination of a problem, it is limited in its ability to identify causal relationships. Despite this limitation, they may help to direct further studies that would establish whether a causal association is present.

Example: psychiatric disorder in women (Dean et al, 1983)

A cross-sectional approach was used to examine psychiatric disorder in women in a community-based sample in Edinburgh. The study had a number of aims, including a comparison of the prevalence of psychiatric illness using a variety of different diagnostic schemes. The schedules involved were the PSE/ID/CATEGO, the SADS/RDC, the Feighner criteria and the Bedford College criteria. The main comparison was made between the PSE and SADS systems and random samples of women from a sector of the city were interviewed using these schedules. The prevalence (both probable and definite cases) for the PSE system was estimated to be 8.7% and for the RDC 13.7%. Although there was a wide discrepancy between these two systems in terms of specific diagnostic labels, the similarity in the overall prevalence rates was good and these rates were comparable with estimations carried out in both Australia and the United States.

Case-control studies

The case-control study is probably the most widely used method to test an aetiological hypothesis. It involves identifying a group of people with a disease or other outcome variable (the cases) and an unaffected group (the controls). The relationship of the aetiological factor or attribute to the disease can be examined by comparing the cases and controls and determing the frequency with which the attribute is present. Case-control studies are usually regarded as retrospective, with both cases and controls identified before the study starts, and the investigator then makes an assessment of the relative importance of the possible causal factors.

Careful consideration must be given to the choice of cases since if generalised statements are to be made about the illness under investigation they must be representative of the group as a whole. To illustrate this, it is known that for a variety of reasons patients referred by their general practitioners to a psychiatric out-patient clinic are not necessarily representative of all cases in the community. This unrepresentativeness is the result of having to pass through a series of 'filters' (Goldberg & Huxley, 1980). A sequence of events takes place which starts with the patient's decision to consult the general practitioner. Patients therefore have to define themselves as ill and then decide that they require professional help. Following this the general practitioner has to diagnose the patients accurately and then consider them appropriate for referral to a specialist. Each of these stages, or filters, is influenced by a variety of factors and awareness of these is essential in the initial selection process.

Similar care must be applied to the selection of controls. Essentially one is comparing a group with an illness or some other variable with a group that does not have that particular illness, in an attempt to identify those factors that are contributing to the pathology. It is essential that these controls come from the same population as the cases and are matched for variables that are considered important. It should be emphasised that once matching is achieved, the effect of the variable used in the match cannot be evaluated as an outcome variable. If a control group is matched, for instance, for age, sex and social class the importance of these variables as aetiological agents can no longer be investigated.

The controls themselves can be selected according to certain strategies, the two most frequently used methods being group and paired controls. In the former case the control group is selected so that it is similar to the study group on the main variables. The degree of matching is dependent upon a combination of the precision that is required and the difficulties associated with selecting such a group. Paired controls involve matching each individual in a study group with a control subject. This method allows for considerably greater precision in matching but is often associated with the practical constraints of finding appropriate subjects.

Care must be taken to ensure that the researcher does not 'overmatch'. In this situation certain variables are matched too closely, with the result that important intermediate variables are obscured.

Cohort studies

Cohort studies are observational and analytical. They involve identifying two or more groups or cohorts of people, who are then followed up for a period of time and compared with each other. The groups must differ in some respect considered important in the natural history of the condition under investigation, because the essential purpose of the study is to assess the outcome of the groups and hence draw conclusions about the relative importance of either the original differences or the experiences in the intervening period. Although usually prospective, the outcome may have already taken place and hence the approach can be seen as retrospective. They are able to provide valuable information on the nature of a relationship and particularly whether there is a causal association. They have one major limitation in that they are often time consuming and expensive, and as a result are usually used only to test specific hypotheses.

Example (Mann et al, 1981)

A representative cohort of patients with non-psychotic psychiatric disorders attending general practitioners were prospectively studied with the aim of identifying those factors important to determining clinical outcome. They demonstrated that the only significant variable to influence the clinical state at the end of the study was the severity of the illness assessed at the outset.

Controlled clinical trials

These may be referred to as intervention studies; they are prospective and experimental and their aim is to determine the effects of a preventive or therapeutic measure on two or more groups of subjects. It is essential that these groups are similar to each other in all respects before the treatment or intervention. Unless this is achieved it will not be possible to conclude from any observed differences that they are the result of the treatment rather than bias. One group is given the treatment or procedure under investigation while the other, the control group, receives a placebo or some alternative known therapeutic measure. The subjects are followed up and after a defined period the outcome is assessed. The conclusions of a clinical trial are based not on individual results but on observed differences in the mean response between the various treatment groups. It is important to be aware that these differences can arise from three possible causes.

(a) *Treatment*: the main objective of the clinical trial has been demonstrated and the treatment or prevention programme has had a genuine effect upon the outcome and is responsible for the observed differences.

(b) *Chance*: differences have been observed but these have occurred by chance in the sample and are not present in the population as a whole. A significance test is used to estimate the likelihood that this has occurred.

(c) *Bias*: the groups differ not only in their response to the treatment but also in some other characteristic and it is this, not the treatment, that is responsible for the observed difference. There are a number of ways that this bias can be avoided or minimised. The patients should be randomly allocated to either the treatment or control group. Any attempts to select the treatment group will inevitably introduce bias. It may be important for both the treatment and control group to believe they are receiving the same therapeutic measure, and so the untreated controls should be given a placebo. Finally both the subjects and the researcher making the outcome assessment may influence the results if they are aware who is receiving the active treatment. For this reason a procedure in which both are deliberately 'blind' to this information should be used (the double-blind trial).

Example: ECT in depression (Freeman et al, 1978)

A double-blind controlled method was used to examine the effectiveness of electroconvulsive therapy (ECT) in the treatment of depressive illness. Forty patients were randomly allocated to one of two groups. The treatment group received bilateral ECT twice weekly, while the control group was given simulated ECT. This simulated ECT involved two 'treatments' in which the electrodes were placed to the patient's head but no current passed. Following this, for the third and subsequent treatments, the group was given normal bilateral ECT. The research worker involved in the clinical assessment at outcome was 'blind' to which patients received either the active or simulated treatments. A number of clinical and self-assessment ratings were completed which confirmed that the clinical state in the treatment group was better than that in the control group. Since all elements of the treatment, apart from the seizure, were identical in the control group, the results supported the suggestion that it was the seizure itself which was the essential therapeutic agent.

Epidemiology and the clinical psychiatrist

It has been suggested that the methods employed in psychiatric epidemiology are of primary importance to the research psychiatrist and the individual responsible for planning the provision of psychiatric health care services. While this is undoubtedly correct it should be emphasised that an understanding of these methods is also of considerable importance to the clinical psychiatrist. This comes from an increasing awareness that the reasoning that lies behind many of the decisions within clinical work involve the counting of clinical events. If valid deductions are to be drawn from these observations then epidemiological methods are required to carry out and analyse this count.

References

BROWN, G. W. & HARRIS, T. (1978) *Social Origins of Depression: A Study of Psychiatric Disorder in Women*. London: Tavistock.

DEAN, C., SURTEES, P. B. & SASHIDHARAN, S. P. (1983) Comparison of research diagnostic systems in an Edinburgh community sample. *British Journal of Psychiatry*, **142**, 247–256.

DYER, J. A. T. & KREITMAN, N. (1984) Hopelessness, depression and suicidal intent in parasuicide. *British Journal of Psychiatry*, **144**, 127–133.

FEIGHNER, J., ROBINS, E., GUZE, S. B., *et al* (1972) Diagnostic criteria for use in psychiatric research. *Archives of General Psychiatry*, **26**, 56–73.

FREEMAN, C. P. C., BASSON, J. V. & CRIGHTON, A. (1978) Double-blind controlled trial of electroconvulsive therapy (ECT) and simulated ECT in depressive illness. *Lancet*, i, 738–740.

GOLDBERG, D. & HUXLEY, P. (1980) *Mental Illness in the Community – The Pathway to Psychiatric Care*. London: Tavistock.

HOLDING, T. A., BUGLASS, D., DUFFY, J. C., *et al* (1977) Parasuicide in Edinburgh – a seven year review 1968–74. *British Journal of Psychiatry*, **130**, 534–543.

INGHAM, J. G. & MILLER, P. (1976) The concept of prevalence applied to psychiatric disorders and symptoms. *Psychological Medicine*, **6**, 217–225.

KENDELL, R. E. (1968) *The Classification of Depressive Illnesses*. Institute of Psychiatry, Maudsley monograph no. 18. London: Oxford University Press.

——, HALL, D. J., HAILEY, A., *et al* (1973) The epidemiology of anorexia nervosa. *Psychological Medicine*, **3**, 200–203.

KREITMAN, N. & DUFFY, J. (1989) Alcoholic and non-alcoholic liver disease in relation to alcohol consumption in Scotland, 1978–84. *British Journal of Addiction* (in press).

LEE, A. S. & MURRAY, R. M. (1988) The long-term outcome of Maudsley depressives. *British Journal of Psychiatry*, **153**, 741–751.

MCMAHON, B. & PUGH, T. F. (1970) *Epidemiology: Principles and Methods*. Boston: Little, Brown & Co.

MANN, A. H., JENKINS, R. & BELSEY, E. (1981) The twelve-month outcome of patients with neurotic illness in general practice. *Psychological Medicine*, **11**, 535–550.

MORRISON, V. L. (1988) Observation and snowballing: useful tools for research into illicit drug use. *Social Pharmacology*, **2**, 247–271.

OFFICE OF POPULATION CENSUSES AND SURVEYS (1986) Occupational mortality 1979–1980, 1982–1983. *Decennial Supplement, Part 1, Commentary*. London: HMSO.

PAYKEL, E. (1980) Recent life events and attempted suicide. In *The Suicide Syndrome* (eds R. Farmer & S. Hirsch). London: Croom Helm.

PLANT, M. A. (1987) *Drugs in Perspective*. London: Hodder & Stoughton.

PRIEST, R. G. (1971) The Edinburgh homeless: a psychiatric survey. *American Journal of Psychotherapy*, **25**, 194–213.

ROSE, G. & BARKER, D. (1979) *Epidemiology for the Uninitiated*. London: British Medical Journal.

SCHLESSELMAN, J. J. (1982) *Case-Control Studies: Design, Conduct, Analysis*. New York: Oxford University Press.

SPITZER, R. L., ENDICOTT, J. & ROBINS, E. (1978) Research Diagnostic Criteria: rationale and reliability. *Archives of General Psychiatry*, **35**, 773–782.

WALTER, S. D. (1978) Calculation of attributable risks from epidemiological data. *International Journal of Epidemiology*, **7**, 179–182.

WALTNER-TOEWS, D. (1982) Nomenclature of risk assessment in 2 × 2 tables. *International Journal of Epidemiology*, **11**, 411–413.

WING, J. K., COOPER, J. E. & SARTORIUS, N. (1974) *The Measurement and Classification of Psychiatric Symptoms*. Cambridge: Cambridge University Press.

—— & STURT, E. (1978) *The PSE-ID-CATEGO System: Supplementary Manual*. London: MRC Social Psychiatry Unit.

Research with single (or few) patients

DAVID F. PECK

There is a long tradition in medicine in general, and in psychiatry in particular, of intensive investigations of single cases. Perhaps the most notable exponent of this was Freud, whose psychoanalytic structure was largely based on detailed clinical observations of a few neurotic patients. Similarly, much of the pioneering work on headache by Wolff and colleagues was based on the intensive investigation of single or just a few cases. Furthermore, many medical journals have regularly published papers based on observations of single or few subjects, for example the *New England Journal of Medicine*, and the *Journal of Nervous and Mental Diseases*.

Although this has often set the scene for important advances, until recently such investigations with small numbers of subjects were often regarded with suspicion. Rigorous experimentalists claim that research with small samples is a throwback to the old mentalist approaches of the Victorian experimental psychologists such as Ebbinghaus, whose enterprise floundered upon the problems of subjectivity, and lack of generalisability to other patients. Edgar & Billingsley (1974) have addressed these issues in some detail.

Over the last decade or so, however, single-case studies have achieved greater acceptability and it is acknowledged that there is no necessary incompatibility between research on small samples and scientific method. A major impetus to this acceptability were the publications by Barlow & Hersen (1973) and Leitenberg (1973), who brought together a series of *experimental* designs that could be applied to single cases or small groups. At the same time, there has been an increasing disenchantment with the methodology (e.g. Candy *et al*, 1972), with the use of statistics (e.g. Gore *et al*, 1977) and with the interpretation and publication of the results (Newcombe, 1987) of usual clinical research involving comparisons of means from large numbers of subjects. A compelling and erudite apology for studying single cases has been given by Bromley (1986), who argues forcefully for the importance of the "case study method". This is "a *quasi judicial* method", which uses "rational argument to interpret empirical evidence" (p. 67) and is concerned with more general issues of working with single cases in a variety of settings.

The focus of the present chapter is much narrower, and concerns simply the single case or experimental designs with small samples. Although many of the single-case experimental designs evolved from within behavioural psychology, it has become increasingly apparent that these methods are more generally applicable in psychiatry (Peck, 1985).

There are several different varieties of experimental design that are appropriate for use with small numbers of subjects. There are no standard procedures, but a series of experimental manipulations all designed to demonstrate a functional relationship between two variables, such as treatment and outcome. Typically this involves systematically altering one variable, and observing its effects on the other. Precisely how this relationship is demonstrated will depend on the characteristics of each clinical situation. As long as this basic logic is followed, it is entirely up to the clinical researcher to use whatever design he feels to be appropriate. Nevertheless for practical purposes, experimental designs with small samples tend to be discussed under two broad headings: ABAB designs, and multiple-baseline designs. With the former, single subjects or single groups of subjects may be used, whereas with the latter it can be appropriate for either single subjects or up to about ten subjects (all with a similar problem). The examples given below are chosen to illustrate the kinds of designs that have been used previously, and the kinds of problems for which they were deemed to be appropriate. One of the main attractions of small samples is that they require a great deal of creativity and ingenuity on the part of researchers to construct an experimental design appropriate to the particular needs.

ABAB designs

This range of designs involves frequent measurement of the patient's problems before, during and after treatment. The period before treatment (baseline or 'A' period) should contain at least two measurement points, but preferably many more. Ideally, baseline measurements should continue until a reasonable degree of stability has been achieved. At that point a treatment (B) is introduced, and the effect on the problem is observed and again measured frequently. When a change has been observed, treatment is discontinued but the problem continues to be measured. If the treatment is responsible for the improvement, then there should be a deterioration at this point. This is the second A or second baseline period. Treatment is then reinstated (second B period), and again an improvement is anticipated (see Fig. 5.1). If there is a clear relationship between when the treatment is applied and an improvement in the clinical problem, one may conclude that the treatment is probably responsible for the change. If, however, similar improvement occurs during the second A phase, then this conclusion would not be warranted. Thus a clear systematic relationship should be demonstrated between the application of treatment, and improvement in

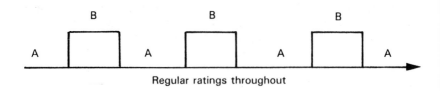

Regular ratings throughout

Fig. 5.1   The extended ABAB design (A = baseline–no treatment, B = treatment intervention)

the patient's problem. The length of the treatment and baseline periods will depend on how quickly the treatment is expected to produce any changes; generally the A and B periods should be of comparable length. Some specific examples of such designs with illustrative clinical applications are detailed below.

The AB design

This is the least convincing of all the single-case designs, because the relationship between treatment application and improvement is observed on only one occasion. Thus there could be many other factors to account for the change in the patient's condition, apart from the initiation of treatment. This may seem but a small improvement upon the gathering of routine clinical data about patients; it is however rather more powerful than this, because of the frequency and systematisation of the measurements of patient problems. This design can be considered when there are good reasons why it would be undesirable to withdraw the treatment and risk deterioration, for example with patients whose condition could be seen as dangerous to themselves or others. The design is strengthened if there is more than one outcome variable and where the baseline period incorporates some form of placebo treatment as a control. A long follow-up period would also be desirable.

Example: Sandman et al *(1987)*

In this study naloxone was used to treat deliberate self-injury in a 21-year-old epileptic woman. In a double-blind AB trial, they administered placebo (saline), followed by three injections of naloxone, in increasing doses. Several outcome measures were used and improvements were obtained in event-related potentials, a memory task, anxiety levels, and frequency of self-injury. Because improvement was not noted during the placebo period, but was after the administration of naloxone, the authors concluded that the drug was responsible for the change.

The ABAB design

As the name suggests, in this design baseline data are recorded, treatment is applied and then withdrawn, and then applied again. Thus a relationship between outcome and treatment intervention is demonstrated on two separate occasions, and this lends more credibility to any conclusions drawn, since alternative explanations of the change, apart from treatment, are less plausible.

Example: de Kock et al *(1984)*

Because of practical constraints, the final design used in this study was not that originally intended by the authors. Nevertheless, some of their data serve as an admirable illustration of the ABAB design. The patient was a severely mentally handicapped woman, aged 32. She exhibited multiple behaviour problems on the ward, involving dressing, washing, toileting, aggression towards other patients and staff, and particularly disruptive behaviour at mealtimes. After baseline measures, the authors adopted the simple but effective technique of instructing a staff member to pay much attention to the patient when she was behaving appropriately at mealtimes, but as far as possible to ignore her when she was behaving inappropriately. The reliability of the observations of her behaviour was assessed by a special observer, and interobserver agreement was consistently above 90%. The results showed a significant improvement upon baseline behaviour, which was reversed when the treatment was withdrawn, but improvement was re-established when treatment was again started. This is a particularly illuminating study since it demonstrates that meaningful data from single cases can be obtained even under difficult clinical circumstances.

More complex AB designs

The basic ABAB format can be extended indefinitely, until the researcher is satisfied that the link between treatment and change has been demonstrated; or the researcher may wish to use any of the many possible variants of this basic design. For example one may wish to compare different dosages or intensities for treatment, as illustrated in the following example.

Example: Hellekson et al *(1986)*

This study was designed to investigate the effectiveness of phototherapy in the treatment of seasonal affective disorder. After obtaining initial assessments of depression using the Hamilton Rating Scale for Depression, they gave phototherapy at three different times of the day (and in this respect could be considered an alternating treatment design– see below), but in each condition the total was two hours per day. Six subjects were involved, and they received the three treatment conditions in a different order. Between each treatment there was a period with no treatment (the A phases). The main finding was that all subjects improved during phototherapy, but this improvement was reversed on each occasion that treatment was withdrawn (Fig. 5.2). There was, however, no difference between the treatments. This study is particularly interesting because it reports a systematic replication using the same method over six subjects, and this adds much credibility to the effectiveness of the treatment. It must be pointed out, however, that because they did not incorporate a placebo treatment, it cannot necessarily be concluded that the light *per se* was responsible for the clinical change.

The alternating treatments design

This design may be used to compare the effects of two or more treatments on one inividual. It comprises rapid and as far as possible random alternation of all the treatments, with an interval between. This design immediately raises questions of interference and carry-over across treatments, but some possible solutions have been suggested: using problems that can be easily reversed; using treatments that have little or no carry-over effect; and finally using some form of sign or cue that is unique to each treatment and salient to the subject.

Example: McGonigle et al *(1987)*

This study was concerned with the treatment of two three-year-old mentally handicapped children. The first patient, a boy, had very poor attention, self-care, and social behaviour; he was also self-injurious. Four methods were used, each with a different cue: they were interruption, differential reinforcement of other behaviour, visual screening, and extinction. It was found that extinction was the most effective and that the differences between treatments were not apparent when there was only a minute between treatments, but were considerably more clear cut when the interval between treatments was 120 minutes. Similar findings were reported with the second child, whose main problems were non-compliance and aggression.

Problems and pitfalls in ABAB designs

At first sight, many of the ABAB designs may seem attractive to the practising clinician, who may consider it feasible to incorporate these research designs into clinical practice without the need for radical change in clinical routine. In reality clinicians may find that the designs are less attractive when they attempt to implement them. There may be reservations concerning the desirability of withdrawing an effective treatment; frequent observations

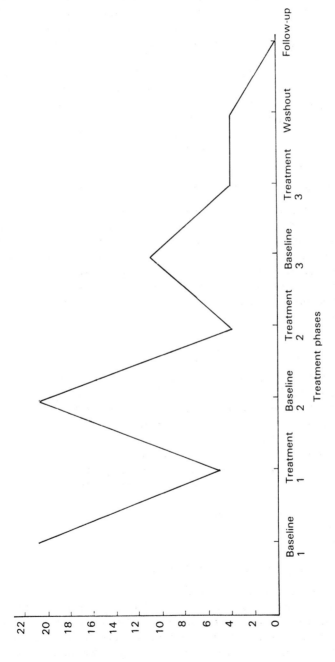

Fig. 5.2   Experimental plot taken from an example of an ABACAD design. The data are from patient 2 in Hellekson et al (1986)

will probably require the co-operation of other staff, which may not be readily achieved; patients may develop another illness and the design may have to be suspended, and so on. In addition it may prove extremely difficult to establish a stable baseline; the outcome measure may not reverse when treatment is withdrawn, particularly if the treatment is especially potent; furthermore the treatment effects may continue for a long time after the treatment has stopped, and so even if the outcome variable is in principle reversible, there may be a long interval between stopping the treatment and the observed change.

For these and other reasons, clinicians may have to content themselves with a simple AB design; that is, systematic and frequent assessment of the problem before treatment, and similar frequent assessments during treatment. Although this design cannot unequivocally demonstrate that the treatment has been effective in a single case, if the same systematic approach is to be adopted with many patients with similar problems, the accumulation in knowledge would be extremely valuable, particularly if the data enabled one to relate patient characteristics to outcome. When confronted with the clinical realities, this may be the most that a clinician can hope for. In many ways of course this is not substantially different from day-to-day good clinical practice and examples abound of systematic clinical observation of a small number of patients producing interesting clinical ideas; for example the report of Wurtman (1985) on the relationship between aspartane and the sudden appearance of epileptic seizures in previously healthy patients.

Other designs

Other alternatives are available to the clinician. For example the repeated pre-test post-test design; this can be used where treatment cannot be administered or withheld at the whim of the researcher, but must be given when required, for example in severe depression. In this design the problem is measured immediately before and immediately after the application of a treatment; if the treatment is effective, the post-treatment measure should regularly be better than the pre-treatment measure. In addition, this design can shed interesting light on the temporal effects of the treatment.

Example: Dykes (1987)

This study was an intensive investigation of the effects of electroconvulsive therapy (ECT) on depression in a series of 12 single cases. Because of the severity of the depression, it was not possible to manipulate the timing of the ECT and it was given as required clinically. Level of depression was assessed before and immediately after each ECT administration. On analysing the data for each patient, it was found that for those who showed an overall good recovery, differences before and after treatment were observed, whereas for patients with poor recovery, changes in depression were unrelated to the timing of the ECT. These trends were apparent on examining the data individually, but would have been obscured if data from all the subjects had been combined for analysis.

The periodic treatments design

Another potentially useful design is for those treatment effects that are not time limited, and may extend into the patient's everyday life; one might anticipate, for example, that the effects of group psychotherapy or social skills training would generalise to the patient's everyday life, and that the patient would continue to improve between attendances. Under these circumstances, the periodic treatments design may be used. It entails providing treatment sessions (preferably at irregular intervals) and frequent monitoring of the patient's progress. If the treatment is effective, there should be an acceleration of progress immediately after each treatment session. In other words there should be more rapid improvement immediately after the treatment session, which should be discernible against a background of gradual improvement.

Conclusion

This is by no means an exhaustive list of the kinds of designs within the overall ABAB format that the clinician may use. The possible designs are limited only by the creativity and ingenuity of the clinician. As long as it can be convincingly demonstrated that there is a relationship between a change in the patient's condition and the application of the treatment, by eliminating or reducing the plausibility of alternative explanations, then the clinician has conformed to the logic behind single-case experimentation.

In addition to the ABAB designs, there is a series of designs that follow a separate logic: the multiple-baseline designs. They are often appropriate when ABAB designs cannot be implemented, for whatever reason; they can also be used with small numbers of patients, as well as single cases.

Multiple-baseline designs

In multiple-baseline designs, several problems or cases are measured simultaneously during a suitable baseline period; subsequently the treatment is applied to one problem, but the other problems continue to be assessed. After a further period the treatment is applied to a second problem (randomly determined) and again all the problems are assessed. Treatment is applied sequentially to each problem in this way, until all the problems have been treated. Thus each problem has a different duration of baseline assessment, which helps to control for 'spontaneous' change. It may be concluded that the treatment has been effective if an improvement is observed in each problem soon after the treatment has been applied; if no improvement is observed, or if one or more of the problems improve before the onset of treatment, then it cannot be concluded that the treatment is responsible for any improvement. This description applies to the multiple baseline across problems; there are also the designs of multiple baseline across subjects (where the same problem is tackled but with different patients) and multiple baseline across settings (where the same problem in the same patient is tackled, but in different settings).

Multiple baseline across problems

Example: Ducker & Moonen (1986)

Three severely mentally handicapped children were the patients in this study; they had no meaningful expressive verbal or non-verbal vocabulary. The authors wished to promote expressive language in the children, using manual signs as the medium of communication. Three different signs were designated for use in the study; those for scissors, mirror, and marbles. The frequency of use of each sign before training was observed for six sessions for 'scissors', after which the expressive language training was started; the frequency of use for 'mirror' was observed for nine baseline sessions before treatment was initiated, and for 'marbles' 14 baseline sessions. There were no recorded observations of any of the three signs before the treatment, but after treatment there was a marked increase. (This is a particularly interesting study from a methodological point of view, since it also incorporated an ABAB component.)

Multiple baseline across subjects

In this design, treatment is applied to several subjects with a similar problem, but after different baseline periods (see Fig. 5.3).

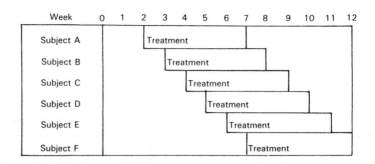

Regular ratings throughout

Fig. 5.3   Multiple-baseline design. Example of six subjects in a trial of five weeks of anxiety management for chronic anxiety as part of a generalised anxiety disorder

Example: Marshall & Peck (1986)

Difficulties in maintaining appropriate facial expressions, and therefore in initiating and maintaining conversation, have been noted in some blind people. The facial expressions of smiling and frowning in five blind adolescents were recorded on videotape before and during training by electromyographic feedback of facial muscle activity. For subject 1 there was one session of baseline recording, after which training was initiated; for subject 2 there were two sessions of baseline, and so on. All videotapes were rated by independent judges, in terms of the naturalness and clarity of the smile and the frown, and of the appropriateness of movements in relevant muscles. Significant improvements were obtained after the initiation of treatment in terms of the smiling, but not the frowning.

Non-current multiple-baseline studies

The design above is useful if all the potential patients are available from the outset. With very rare conditions this may not be the case, and it would not be feasible or ethical to delay treatment for some patients until five or six with a similar problem have been referred. Under these circumstances it is possible to carry out a 'non-current' multiple-baseline study, in which the durations of the baselines are specified in advance for as many patients as are expected, and one of these durations is randomly selected as each patient is referred.

Multiple baseline across settings

Treatment is applied to a particular problem with a patient, in one particular setting; the same problem is also measured in different settings, but treatment is not applied. Sometime afterwards, the treatment is applied in the second setting and so on until treatment has been applied across all the settings. This design is infrequently used, since it assumes that the improvement in one setting will not generalise to the other settings involved; there will be few clinical problems where this obtains.

Example: Odom et al *(1985)*

In this study three mentally handicapped boys were taught to increase the frequency of social interactions, such as demonstrating affection, sharing things with other children, and helping children. These social skills were initiated by other, non-handicapped children, who had previously been trained to initiate social interactions by teachers. The training took place across three classroom settings, in sequential order. A marked improvement in social interaction was observed, but only when it was applied in each setting individually.

ation of results

It _ _ditional in group experimental studies to use inferential statistics, such as *t*-tests and analysis of variance, to help decide whether a treatment is effective. It has been argued that in research with small samples, because each subject is assessed so frequently and intensively, treatment effects are normally quite clear cut, and statistical techniques to help in making decisions are not necessary; if statistical analysis is needed to tease out an effect, the effect cannot be of large magnitude in the first place, and may therefore be irrelevant for practical clinical purposes.

To some research workers, such notions may be appealing. On the other hand, others have argued that using visual inspection of the data alone can lead to major errors, and therefore that statistical analysis is necessary. Under most circumstances, it would appear that one does in fact come to the same conclusions using either statistical analysis or visual inspection. However, there are some circumstances, particularly where there is a trend in the baseline data, where discrepancies may occur. The wary research worker is, therefore, best advised to use some form of statistical analysis to supplement decisions.

Unfortunately, for technical statistical reasons, the data from the simplest of experimental designs (e.g. AB designs) require the most complex of statistical procedures for analysis (e.g. transfer function analysis). Such methods require sophisticated computer facilities, and a large number of observations, probably over 50. For these and other reasons, such analyses are unlikely to appeal to most clinical researchers. However, some simpler alternatives have recently been advocated; these have been well described by Morley & Adams (1989) to which the reader is urged to turn.

Conclusions

Study designs with small samples appear to have many advantages: few subjects are required; matched control groups are not necessary; scientifically acceptable research can be fitted in with everyday practice; and inferential statistics *may* (although this is not advised) be avoided. On the other hand, there are several problems and pitfalls in the use of these designs, already alluded to.

Small samples should not be seen only as alternatives to large-scale group studies, but as complementary to them; interesting hypotheses may emerge that warrant a larger-scale trial, and data from patients within a large trial can be examined individually, giving a more accurate indication of variation in response to treatment.

It is important to reiterate that a 'cook-book' approach to such research is not appropriate. The design should be tailored according to the circumstances of the particular patients and problems. As Hayes (1981) has argued, what is required in single-case research is "an attitude of investigative play", rather than slavish adherence to a fixed design; he goes on to describe various ways in which experimental designs can be adapted to meet clinical constraints.

It is also important to emphasise that there is little that is new or different about these designs as such. There are many examples (e.g. McPherson & Le Gassicke, 1965; Stabenau *et al*, 1970) of psychiatric research utilising precursors of small-sample designs. Furthermore, the authors of several of the examples given in this chapter (e.g. Hellekson *et al*, 1986; Sandman *et al*, 1987) did not explicitly term their studies small-sample designs; they simply devised an experimental design to answer specific questions, and the design that resulted followed the appropriate logic. It could also be argued that using small-sample designs hardly differs from current notions of good clinical practice. What is new and different is that varying approaches to such research have been brought together to form a coherent approach to research methodology, a coherence that has led to an increasing scientific acceptability. Psychiatric research would probably gain much from wider use of research with small samples.

References

BARLOW, D. & HERSEN, M. (1973) Single-case experimental designs: uses in applied clinical research. *Archives of General Psychiatry*, **29**, 319–325.

BROMLEY, D. (1986) *The Case-Study Method in Psychology and Related Disciplines*. Chichester: Wiley.

CANDY, J., BALFOUR, F. H. G., CAWLEY, R. H., *et al* (1972) A feasibility study for a controlled trial of formal psychotherapy. *Psychological Medicine*, **2**, 345–362.

DE KOCK, U., MANSELL, J., FELCE, D., *et al* (1984) Establishing appropriate mealtime behaviour of a severely disruptive mentally handicapped woman. *Behavioural Psychotherapy*, **12**, 163–174.

DUCKER, P. C. & MOONEN, X. M. (1986) The effect of procedures on spontaneous signing with Down's syndrome children. *Journal of Mental Deficiency Research*, **30**, 355–364.

DYKES, S. R. (1987) *Process of Change in Mood and Cognition During a Course of Electroconvulsive Therapy*. MPhil. thesis, University of Edinburgh.

EDGAR, E. & BILLINGSLEY, F. (1974) Believability when $N = 1$. *Psychological Record*, **24**, 147–160.

GORE, S. M., JONES, I. G. & RYTTER, E. C. (1977) Misuse of statistical methods: critical assessment of articles in BMJ from January to March, 1976. *British Medical Journal*, **i**, 85–87.

HAYES, S. C. (1981) Single case experimental design and empirical clinical practice. *Journal of Consulting and Clinical Psychology*, **49**, 193–211.

HELLEKSON, C. J., KLINE, J. A. & ROSENTHAL, N. E. (1986) Phototherapy for seasonal affective disorder in Alaska. *American Journal of Psychiatry*, **143**, 1035–1037.

LEITENBERG, H. (1973) The use of single-case methodology in psychotherapy research. *Journal of Abnormal Psychology*, **82**, 87–101.

MARSHALL, M. J. & PECK, D. F. (1986) Facial expression training in blind adolescents using EMG feedback: a multiple-baseline study. *Behaviour Research and Therapy*, **24**, 429–435.

MCGONIGLE, J. J., ROJAHN, J., DIXON, J., *et al* (1987) Multiple treatment interference in the alternating treatments design as a function of the intercomponent interval length. *Journal of Applied Behavior Analysis*, **20**, 171–178.

MCPHERSON, F. M. & LE GASSICKE, J. (1965) A single-patient self-controlled and self-recorded trial of Wy 3498. *British Journal of Psychiatry*, **111**, 149–154.

MORLEY, S. & ADAMS, M. (1989) Some simple statistical tests for exploring single case time series data. *British Journal of Social and Clinical Psychology* (in press).

NEWCOMBE, R. G. (1987) Towards a reduction in publication bias. *British Medical Journal*, **295**, 656–659.

ODOM, S. L., HOYSON, M., JAMIESON, B., *et al* (1985) Increasing handicapped preschoolers' peer/social interactions: cross setting and component analysis. *Journal of Applied Behavior Analysis*, **18**, 3–16.

PECK, D. F. (1985) Small *N* research in clinical practice. In *New Developments in Clinical Psychology* (ed. F. Watts). London: Wiley.

SANDMAN, C. A., BARRON, J. L., COINELLA, F. M., *et al* (1987) Influence of naloxone on brain and behavior of a self-injurious woman. *Biological Psychiatry*, **22**, 899–906.

STABENAU, J. R., CREVELING, C. R. & DALEY, J. (1970) The 'pink spot', 3,4-dimethoxyphenylethylamine, common tea and schizophrenia. *American Journal of Psychiatry*, **127**, 611–616.

WURTMAN, R. J. (1985) Aspartane: possible effect on seizure susceptibility. *Lancet*, *ii*, 1060.

Further reading

BARLOW, D. H. & HERSEN, M. (1984) *Single Case Experimental Designs* (2nd edn). New York: Pergamon.

KAZDIN, A. (1982) *Single Case Research Designs: Methods for Clinical and Applied Settings*. New York: Oxford University Press.

MORLEY, S. (1988) Single case research. In *Handbook of Research in Clinical Psychology* (eds F. Watts & G. Parry). Brighton: Erlbaum.

6 Research in psychotherapy

FRANK MARGISON and GRAEME McGRATH

Research in psychotherapy has a bad reputation, and has also had a bad press (*Lancet*, 1984; Wilkinson, 1984; Shepherd, 1984). The purpose of this chapter is to face two of the sources of this notoriety. First is the assumption by other researchers that psychotherapy research is either not done at all or done badly. Without special pleading we shall show that by its very nature psychotherapy research produces particular difficulties, both conceptual and practical. However, in overcoming such difficulties psychotherapy researchers have advanced methodology in ways which could usefully be incorporated into project designs in other areas of psychiatry.

The second reason for notoriety follows from the first. Good research advisers will often tell beginners to steer well clear of psychotherapy research, particularly for small-scale projects that are to be requirements for MSc or MPhil degree dissertations or their equivalent, because the cost of overcoming many of the inherent problems in outcome research is so great. The traditional alternative was to escape into 'process' research, which can be divorced from clinical reality if the principle of linking process with outcome becomes obscured.

A third issue is the regular claim (e.g. Shepherd, 1984) that psychotherapy has no significant treatment effect, but research has frequently shown significant effects for a wide variety of psychotherapy methods and these issues have been widely debated elsewhere (e.g. Garfield & Bergin, 1978, 1986; Bloch & Lambert, 1985; McGrath & Lowson, 1987).

Particular difficulties in psychotherapy research

Many reviewers (Gottman & Markman, 1978; Crown, 1981; American Psychiatric Association, 1982; Bloch, 1985; Gomes-Schwartz, 1982; Kazdin, 1986) have outlined the particular difficulties of psychotherapy research. They are summarised briefly below, under separate headings.

Psychotherapy treatments are difficult to define and operationalise

Herink (1980) defined 250 different psychotherapy treatment approaches. This diversity has led to a prolific number of small studies on non-standardised and often non-comparable populations. Even with relatively common treatment strategies such as desensitisation there can be important differences in the precise components of the treatment.

In an attempt to clarify this model it is now necessary to specify treatment *purity* and treatment *distinctness* in outcome studies. Treatment 'purity' is analogous to the specificity of pharmacological effects of a drug. Simply, it is the extent to which a treatment is homogeneous across sessions and across therapists, while already being consistent with a specified model (ideally one that is closely linked to a particular theoretical framework).

Major efforts have been made to 'manualise' therapies, with handbooks that specify the ways in which a therapist should behave within a particular treatment mode and in response to particular clinical situations. Simple manuals have been developed for prescriptive therapy and exploratory therapy in the Sheffield study (Shapiro & Firth, 1987). Much more complex manuals were developed for the Depression Collaborative Study at the National Institute of Mental Health (NIMH) (Waskow, 1984). Even when treatments are specified, good design requires therapists to be trained in particular techniques and for some form of monitoring of treatment in order to maintain treatment consistency.

Treatment 'distinctness' refers to the extent to which the treatments to be compared can be differentiated. If two treatments are compared using small samples and they appear to be equally effective, this may be a statistical error due to the inability of the experimental conditions to distinguish significant differences between treatments. In other words, the small sample size means that the study did not have sufficient power to detect a difference between treatments even though one actually exists (see Chapter 2). If one treatment is known to be effective then the other may wrongly be deemed equally effective because of this type II error.

'Control groups' and 'placebo' present difficulties conceptually and practically

This is especially true when 'non-specific' treatment effects tend to obscure specific effects. Even 'waiting-list' controls have to have initial contact and evaluation. In psychotherapy these initial contacts have sufficient in common with the formation of a treatment contract to contaminate severely controls for the initial evaluations of treatment. In retrospect many treated patients having received an explanation about the trial, to fulfil ethical requirements, date the onset of hopeful expectations about treatment to the first contact, not to the first session, hence blurring the specific treatment effects. Malan *et al* (1975) produced evidence that for some patients significant changes can occur after an assessment session alone. In addition, a true placebo control is difficult to imagine. Paul (1966), in a key study on desensitisation, provided an excellent and plausible 'attention' placebo by giving a placebo 'tranquilliser' plus a plausible rationale for carrying out a cognitive task as a believable alternative treatment.

Disturbingly for the whole basis of psychotherapy research, such plausible placebos given convincingly have highly significant treatment effects. These often have clear links with the effective components of other psychotherapeutic methods, implying a set of 'non-specific' treatment factors common to many forms of psychotherapy. To compound this confusion, in comparative studies it has been shown by meta-analysis that the treatment most favoured by the investigators tends to have significant advantages irrespective of the treatment type (Kazdin, 1986). The whole notion of non-specific treatment effects has been rethought as a result of these difficulties (e.g. Shapiro, 1984), so that for example the active (or veridical) treatment condition in one study could be used in another study as an 'attention control'. Hence, the simple notion of 'placebo controlled' as applied to physical treatment trials may be inappropriate in psychotherapy research design.

With small sizes of specific treatment effect, large samples are needed

Large samples are needed to obtain sufficient power to detect differences between treatments. If even sophisticated studies by seasoned researchers present difficulties of treatment equivalence in control comparison studies, small-scale researchers will be unable to generate sufficient numbers to provide statistical power adequate to discriminate effectively between similar treatments. Power calculations in this situation are crucial to avoid meaningless 'no significant differences' between results (see Chapter 2).

Measures of outcome are often 'soft' and choice of measures is critical

Multiple measures of outcome are often needed. Waskow & Parloff (1975) suggested the use of an outcome measures 'battery' covering (a) objective measures (i.e. by observer), (b) self-report measures, (c) standardised diagnostic and symptomatic measures and (d) measures as specific as possible to the treatment being evaluated.

No equivalent updated battery has been produced that has been accepted in the UK, but most researchers do follow the principles outlined above in selecting measures of outcome. However, there is a problem in knowing which measures to see as reflecting improvement most accurately. A psychodynamic psychotherapist would probably say that a higher weighting should be given to measures of dynamic change, as shown in relationships, self-esteem, and social functioning (Malan *et al*, 1975), whereas a behaviourally orientated researcher would give priority to improvements in specified target behaviour.

Even in well designed studies it is difficult to generalise to routine clinical populations

Even if all the above complex issues are resolved, there remains the difficulty that researchers usually aim to treat patients drawn from specific diagnostic or symptomatic groups (e.g. major depression as defined by Research Diagnostic Criteria).

Elliott (1983) has drawn attention to the lack of response by clinicians to clear research results apparently relevant to their favoured modes of treatment. Partly this can be understood as a consequence of research being in the main carried out by a different group of clinicians from those in full-time clinical practice. In addition, the need to research 'pure' groups makes it difficult to generalise results to the more 'fuzzy' diagnostic groups in unselected clinical practice. Finally, it is likely that delivering new forms of treatment in response to research results may require the development of new skills on the part of the clinician. This is clearly different from the effect that a treatment trial of a new drug might have on clinical practice.

Treatment evaluation strategies

Kazdin (1986) has summarised the treatment evaluation strategies relevant to psychotherapy design. These can be seen as different ways of dividing the 'packages' characteristically offered during psychotherapy.

Treatment package strategy

A whole treatment package, containing a variety of elements, which may be individually effective, is evaluated. For example, many interventions that can be seen under the broad heading of psychosocial treatments for cancer patients are initially investigated without subdivision (e.g. Gordon *et al*, 1980; Maguire *et al*, 1980). This approach has the advantage of keeping within existing mixed clinical practice but with the obvious disadvantage of not knowing which precise intervention contributes most to the eventual outcome.

Dismantling strategy

The next step after a package has been shown to be effective is to separate particular components, with some patients receiving the whole package and some the package minus one or more of these specific parts.

The approach has an inherent logic that has been highly effective in improving and often simplifying treatment approaches, particularly in behavioural therapy (e.g. for desensitisation compared to exposure (Kazdin & Wilcoxon, 1976)) but is limited to treatments that can be broken into discrete and specifiable segments. Some components, particularly in the interpersonal and exploratory modes of therapy, while being specifiable in principle, are very difficult to remove without the treatment seeming arbitrary and bizarre. For example, the removal of all empathy would lead to an extraordinary therapeutic style. The alternative, where a particular parameter is offered in different 'strengths', is discussed under the heading 'Parametric', below.

Constructive approach

This is the opposite approach, where components are added and evaluated sequentially, preferably to an already proven treatment. An example would be adding cognitive or dynamic psychotherapies to pharmacological treatments (Weissman (1979) reviews a number of such studies).

Example (Weissman et al, 1979)

In a randomised controlled trial male and female patients aged 18–65 and satisfying DSM–III (American Psychiatric Association, 1980) criteria for major depressive disorder were allocated to four treatment groups. One group received short-term interpersonal psychotherapy, another amitriptyline, a third group a combination of psychotherapy and pharmacotherapy and a final 'control' group had no active treatment but were able to contact the therapist as required. Outcome, measured as symptomatic improvement, showed no difference between psychotherapy and pharmacotherapy, but a clear difference in favour of the combination of both.

Again the approach has a pleasing logic which is difficult to apply in actual research, and a strategy that is feasible in a structured research protocol may lead to confusion when a clinician tries to use similar combinations in an uncontrolled clinical setting.

Parametric

This approach is suitable for systematic refinement of an existing treatment by careful alteration of the degree or intensity of a measurable component which however remains present in all experimental conditions. Good examples can be found in the behavioural research literature.

Example (Stern & Marks, 1973)

A group of chronically agoraphobic patients were treated by exposure ('flooding') to the most feared situation, with two sessions of short exposure and two sessions of longer exposure, in random order. Each treatment session began with exposure in fantasy followed by exposure in real life. Long exposure was superior in both fantasy and reality, and all significant treatment effects favoured long exposure in reality. This had significant implications for clinical practice, and now most treatment programmes for agoraphobia adopt this style of management.

This strategy is particularly effective in psychotherapy research where a component can be operationally defined. However, it is easy to fall into the error of making *post-hoc* divisions of therapies into 'high' and 'low' on a particular parameter and assuming that these offer the same distinction between treatments as when these separations are made prospectively and carried through purposefully by a clinician who has some knowledge of the study design. *Post-hoc* analysis is of some use in generating hypotheses for further evaluation but must be distinguished from a planned application of different levels of a particular treatment parameter.

It may also be extremely difficult to change only one parameter without influencing others. For example, studies that have led to a decrease in 'closed questions' by therapists tend to show the therapists compensating by increasing other particular types of interventions (Goldberg *et al*, 1984).

Comparative treatment strategies

This is the design most familiar to researchers in physical treatments. To date most psychotherapy studies have yielded disappointing results when following this strategy. This is often called the 'treatment equivalence paradox' (Stiles *et al*, 1986) – the harder you try to separate modes of therapy the more they seem to resemble each other in terms of outcome. Luborsky *et al* (1975) compared this with the caucus race from *Alice* – "all have won and all shall have prizes".

Example (Waskow, 1984)

The American NIMH has been involved in a multicentre comparative study of different forms of psychotherapy for depression. In this study three types of treatment are compared – cognitive therapy, interpersonal therapy, and clinical management (a standardised approach to pharmacotherapy), including placebo. Treatments are specified in manual form, training and supervision are by experts in the respective treatments and treatment integrity will be assessed at the end of the study. Although the outcome data have not yet been published, the results should give valuable information about which therapies work best with which individuals, and whether specific therapy techniques are more effective than 'non-specific' factors common to all treatment.

Comparative designs have particular problems because of difficulties in keeping treatments distinct, offering optimal 'dosages' for each treatment, and keeping other variables constant across treatments. However, these designs can yield fascinating findings on close examination even when treatment effects are only broadly comparable. For example Weissman *et al* (1979) in their study of interpersonal therapy versus pharmacotherapy found roughly comparable treatment outcomes but different *profiles* of improvement consistent with each treatment offered. This suggests that behind the apparent treatment equivalence there may be different change processes occurring that are different for each treatment approach.

Process research strategies

Modern research design has shifted towards combining process research measures, for example Stiles' (1979) session evaluation questionnaire, which systematically measures the client's experience of a session in terms of 'smoothness' and 'depth' against outcome measures assessed at the same time. The disadvantage of such measures is that they generally involve both patient and therapist in long and complex analyses of sessions conducted by independent assessors, and thus require a considerable investment of time and money. Detailed studies of process can generate clinical hypotheses about the processes of change obscured in the 'treatment equivalence paradox'.

Client and therapist variation strategies

Many attempts have been made to examine systematically the effects of fixed characteristics of therapist and patient such as age, race and sex, individual characteristics, such as credibility or attractiveness, and therapist variables, such as genuineness, empathy, and non-possessive warmth (for reviews see Garfield, 1986; Beutler *et al*, 1986). Lambert *et al* (1983) suggested that variables rated highly by patients may contribute a significant amount to outcome variance. These parameters have been widely studied in psychotherapy research but almost totally neglected in the delivery of physical treatments where such variance is seen as 'noise' in the experimental system.

Combined strategies

The above strategies can be linked in an outcome study, for example in a large comparison study of two treatments. In such a study clients can be so recruited as to allow systematic comparisons at the same time of client and therapist variables such as age, sex, race, etc., to measure the interactions of these variables with the main treatment effect variables.

The 'best available' strategies

From the critical approach to design problems inherent in psychotherapy research several issues have been tackled that have implications for psychiatric research in other clinical areas.

(a) In the NIMH Depression Collaborative Study (Waskow, 1984) great attention was paid to the way in which drugs/placebo were delivered in the active drug and placebo conditions. Detailed manuals specified how much time and advice should be given by the medical attendant, how much reassurance should be given and how it should be given, and other ways of optimising drug delivery were outlined. This approach could be easily applied in main-stream pharmacological studies with the likely effect of reducing spurious variance due to the conditions under which the drug was delivered. In addition these methods offer a good model of medical practice, drawing from available literature for strategies to maximise compliance and the treatment alliance.

(b) Recruitment to treatment groups can be stratified to measure interaction effects of treatment with other variables known to influence outcome such as specific patient and therapist variables.

(c) Attempts have been made when 'manualising' many treatments to produce acceptable training packages that allow inexperienced clinicians to master the necessary skills as quickly as possible while maximising the homogeneity of the treatment approach. The Conversational Model (Hobson, 1985) was an attempt to delineate a complex exploratory mode of therapy (Maguire *et al*, 1984) sufficiently to allow the basics to be taught quickly and efficiently (Goldberg *et al*, 1984) and then to generalise this teaching to other departments using videotape teaching methods (Margison & Hobson, 1983). Trainees greatly appreciate such simple models of practice which reduce anxieties about beginning therapy while allowing them to discuss the necessary uncertainties of practice in psychotherapy in the more focused supervision which ensues.

The benefits and limitations of the double-blind controlled trial (the 'drug design paradigm') have been extensively discussed elsewhere (Orlinsky & Howard, 1986). There has been a sharpening of the questions about group comparisons to measure outcome in the last two decades as sophisticated methods of design and data analysis have been introduced. While there is still a place for such design in large-scale psychotherapy research projects, researchers have also led the way in introducing alternative research methods.

Alternative approaches

Example (Freeman et al, *1988)*

In a trial of psychotherapy for bulimia nervosa both restricted randomisation and stratification were used. The study compared behaviour therapy, cognitive behaviour therapy and group therapy for bulimia. To avoid subjects who were randomly allocated to group treatment having to wait much longer for therapy while a group was collected, the ratio of randomisation was altered in favour of group treatment a few weeks before a new group was going to start. Allocation was still entirely random, but more than a third of subjects were allocated to group therapy. To control for therapist variables the two therapists each treated half the behaviour therapy patients and half the cognitive therapy patients, and they combined to carry out group treatment. Stratification was used to ensure that equal numbers of severely disordered patients were allocated to each group.

Several developments in psychotherapy research have provided new opportunities for small-scale research projects. Four different alternative methods of research design are mentioned briefly in this section:

(a) single case study designs
(b) process outcome research
(c) use of 'hard' measures of outcome
(d) techniques of meta-analysis.

These strategies for research offer advantages for clinicians daunted by the inherent difficulties of much outcome research.

Single case study designs

Some of the most useful developments from behavioural psychotherapy research are the methods that allow a researcher with limited resources to make systematic statements about treatment effects on samples as small as one patient. This method clearly has much to offer the small-scale researcher (Kazdin, 1986). Peck (1985; see also Chapter 5) describes briefly the basic design issues. He points out that few researchers have used single case study methodology other than for strictly defined target behaviour within a strict behavioural treatment method. In principle, however, the design could be applied using measures more appropriate for assessing change in dynamic psychotherapy.

Single-case experiments utilise the patient as his/her own control. Some conditions are therefore desirable.

(a) There must be a sufficiently long lead-in to assess baseline status.
(b) The measures should be as clear as possible and directly measurable at the end of each session and preferably every day.
(c) The treatment, ideally, should permit periods on and off treatment without making nonsense of the treatment approach.

These permit ABABA-type designs. Unfortunately this also makes such research particularly difficult in psychodynamic therapies because of the unlikelihood of linear change following treatment, compared with the relatively direct, specific and readily measurable impacts of a behavioural approach. Indeed, Shapiro & Hobson (1972) showed some evidence for immediate *worsening* after sessions of exploratory therapy despite long-term benefits, a finding of great interest in itself.

(d) The goals of therapy must be defined particularly clearly with plausible measures of change available.

Example (Kandel et al, *1977; cited in Kazdin, 1986)*

An autistic boy spent much of his time at his special school withdrawn and talking to himself. Treatment to improve social interaction consisted of demonstrating appropriate social behaviours, followed by the introduction of two children who were rewarded with sweets for playing with the boy. This treatment was introduced for a series of sessions at one time in the school day, and then changed to a different time. In each case measured social interaction improved following a period of systematic exposure. This improvement was maintained on six-month follow-up.

A particular benefit of this approach is that "it reduces the hiatus between research and practice, and researcher and practitioner" (Kazdin, 1986). It has been conventional to avoid using tests of statistical significance to measure the reliability of changes in outcome measures when using single case study designs. The underlying assumption is that differences that are not immediately obvious and clearly related to the start and cessation of the active treatment are likely to be of limited clinical relevance. However, methods of data analysis are available that take account of this (reviewed in Kazdin, 1986).

The approach could be criticised from the standpoint of the drug trial paradigm on several grounds:

(a) lack of external control groups
(b) lack of blindness
(c) small sample sizes
(d) lack of generalisability to large clinical populations.

These points have led to single case study methodology being compared to phase I trials of new drugs. This seriously underestimates the possible impacts of this research.

(a) The methodology allows individualised measures of change that are very difficult to apply in designs comparing group means (although the Personal Questionnaire Rapid Scaling Technique is an attempt to overcome this (Mulhall, 1976)).

(b) Results that are more systematic than the usual anecdotal case reports can be obtained in rare conditions.

(c) The method can be applied widely in clinical practice itself (the so-called 'quasi-experimental approach').

(d) The method can generate further clinical hypotheses about points of change.

(e) The method, by using the patient as his/her own control, over-comes some of the inherent difficulties in obtaining adequate control groups.

(f) The opportunity to do a series of comparable single case studies over a period of time allows clinical practitioners to study treatment effects in reasonably large numbers of patients.

Process outcome research

These approaches were described briefly above as strategies in large-scale outcome research. Here two recent techniques are outlined that can be used intensively to study 'change' events in therapy.

Interpersonal recall (IPR) was originally developed as a teaching method (Kagan, 1980). Briefly, the approach is to replay tapes of sessions to the client and/or therapist to identify key points in sessions. Elliott (1985) has developed a technique for generating rich and detailed accounts in a subsequent semistructured interview with the client. The method has been used to complement large-scale outcome methods but could be used as a clinically sensitive tool more widely. There are obvious disadvantages in that the method could potentially interfere with the therapy by, in effect, having a replay session with commentary before the next session. In addition recall of sessions may not accurately reflect the experience of the session itself. However, the method has the advantage of retaining the richness and emphasis on direct experience of the therapeutic process itself and is therefore particularly good for developing specific hypotheses for further research or, in its own right, offering an 'inner eye' onto the private world of therapy.

An extension of this method called Comprehensive Process Analysis (CPA; Elliott, 1985) uses a group of clinicians to study all the information about a particularly salient event in therapy. The research group tries to achieve consensus about a plausible pathway by which antecedent factors (e.g. symptoms; age, sex and background of therapist and client; social context; etc.) lead to events before the session, thence to events within the session, and finally to the point in therapy to be studied. A detailed description of this event leads to an account of short-term and longer-term influences and impacts. By developing several of these putative mechanisms of change, the clinical experience of the researchers is dovetailed with the direct experience of the therapist and client which again produces clinically rich and systematic accounts of therapeutic effects. This is not only a new paradigm for research, but provides the opportunity to clarify what may be important elements in the process of psychotherapy, which in turn can feed into other research models.

Use of 'hard' measures of outcome

A very different strategy is to borrow measures of outcome from the rest of general medicine and surgery. The method is limited to particular situations such as liaison practice, where a psychotherapy intervention can be used with a defined group of patients where clearly defined measures of outcome are also available. Naturally, other measures of psychological and social change are usually included in the study design. Fairburn *et al* (1986) treated patients with bulimia nervosa and included weight gain and menstrual function as 'hard' measures of change.

Similar strategies are beginning to be used in patients with physical illnesses. Rosser *et al* (1983) used this strategy when measuring forced expiratory volume (FEV_1) as an outcome measure in patients with chronic obstructive airways disease. A similar approach currently in progress (Ryle & Hilton, unpublished) uses glycosylated haemoglobin (a measure of blood glucose stability) to assess the stability of 'brittle' diabetics before, during and after a brief structured therapeutic intervention. Both of these studies have particularly relevant and plausible outcome measures. However, even 'hard' measures show considerable individual variance, and such measures as tumour staging, while theoretically of relevance, are more applicable to large-scale outcome studies, as the predicted effects of therapy would require large sample sizes to have sufficient power to give reliable results.

The main requirements are an accessible clinical population, good co-operation with surgical and medical colleagues, and an available and relevant measure of change. Such studies make a plausible case that research strategies can go beyond the common 'defensive' approach adopted by researchers who merely ask whether psychotherapy can do 'as well as' other interventions such as tricyclic antidepressants.

Techniques of meta-analysis

An approach to reviewing the literature rather than 'hands on' research, this technique has become popular recently despite criticisms from some researchers (Eysenck, 1983; Shepherd, 1984). In the psychiatric literature this method has been used particularly in psychotherapy research (Smith & Glass, 1977). A collection of outcome studies is taken (the initial selection being critical (Shapiro & Shapiro, 1982)) and subjected to systematic review of relevant variables (e.g. sample size, treatment methods used). A mathematical technique is then used to adjust measures of change so that studies can, in principle, be compared numerically with each other. The difference between treated and untreated controls is measured in units equivalent to the size of the standard deviation of the control group. This method has generally confirmed the 'treatment equivalence paradox' mentioned above but has provided some surprises. Shapiro & Shapiro (1982) reported, for example, the counterintuitive result that the research on psychodynamic psychotherapy was generally at a higher level of methodological sophistication than the group of studies on behavioural methods.

Meta-analysis should not, however, be seen as a 'soft' alternative to clinical research. The methodology is complex and fraught with difficulty (Shapiro & Shapiro, 1983; Kazdin, 1986) – it is not merely a brief literature review. Considerable ground knowledge of psychotherapy research techniques is the minimum requirement for any researcher considering a meta-analytic study.

Conclusion

Psychotherapy research presents particular challenges, but in the attempt to tackle complex methodological problems new approaches are being developed which are near to the experience of clinicians while being systematic. Some of these new approaches have the added advantage, outlined above, of being particularly suitable for clinician researchers with limited resources. This chapter has reviewed some of the difficulties inherent in psychotherapy research design and outlined some of the many alternative approaches available. We have implicitly adopted the view that much current medical research uses strategies inappropriate to the practice of psychotherapy. Plum (1981) criticises the technological ideology prevalent in current research, stating that it places "skilfulness instead of meaning at the heart of personal communication", with the risk that the therapist may end up, in the phrase of Krasner (1962), as merely a "social reinforcement machine".

The unfortunate polarisation across a classical versus romantic dimension has blocked psychotherapy research much more effectively than any problems inherent in psychotherapy research design. Even if researchers show clear differences in outcome, in the climate described above they are unlikely to influence clinical practice. A way through this is for clinicians to see research as being clinically relevant and an acceptable part of their own practice. In psychotherapy, research should also reflect, at least in part, the complexity inherent in a treatment which is defined as having a relationship central to the method itself (Brown & Pedder, 1979; Storr, 1979).

References

AMERICAN PSYCHIATRIC ASSOCIATION (1980) *Diagnostic and Statistical Manual of Mental Disorders* (3rd edn) (DSM–III). Washington, DC: APA.
—— (1982) *Psychotherapy Research: Methodological and Efficiency Issues.* American Psychiatric Association Commission on the Psychotherapies. Washington, DC: APA.

BEUTLER, L. E., CRAGO, M. & ARIZMENDI, T. G. (1986) Research on therapist variables in psychotherapy. In *Handbook of Psychotherapy and Behaviour Change* (3rd edn) (eds S. L. Garfield & A. E. Bergin), pp. 257–310. New York: John Wiley.

BLOCH, S. (1985) Psychotherapy. In *Recent Advances in Clinical Psychiatry*, vol. 4. (ed. K. Granville-Grossman). London: Churchill Livingstone.

—— & LAMBERT, M. J. (1985) What price psychotherapy? A rejoiner. *British Journal of Psychiatry*, **146**, 96–98.

BROWN, D. & PEDDER, J. (1979) *Introduction to Psychotherapy*. London: Tavistock.

CROWN, S. (1981) Psychotherapy research today. *British Journal of Hospital Medicine*, **25**, 492–502.

ELLIOTT, R. (1983) Fitting process research to the practising psychotherapist. *Psychotherapy: Theory, Research and Practice*, **20**, 47–55.

—— (1985) Helpful and non-helpful events in brief counselling interviews: an empirical taxonomy. *Journal of Consulting and Clinical Psychology*, **32**, 307–321.

EYSENK, H. J. (1983) Special review of M. L. Smith, G. V. Glass and T. L. Miller: the benefits of psychotherapy. *Behaviour Research and Therapy*, **21**, 315–320.

FAIRBURN, C. G., KIRK, J., O'CONNOR, M., *et al* (1986) A comparison of 2 psychological treatments for bulimia nervosa. *Behaviour Research and Therapy*, **24**, 629–644.

FREEMAN, C. P., BARRY, F., DUNKELD-TURNER, J., *et al* (1988) A controlled trial of psychotherapy for bulimia nervosa. *British Medical Journal*, **296**, 521–525.

GARFIELD, S. L. (1986) Research on client variables in psychotherapy. *Handbook of Psychotherapy and Behaviour Change* (3rd edn) (eds S. L. Garfield & A. E. Bergin), pp. 213–256. New York: John Wiley.

—— & BERGIN, A. E. (eds) (1978) *Handbook of Psychotherapy and Behaviour Change* (2nd edn). New York: John Wiley.

—— & —— (eds) (1986) *Handbook of Psychotherapy and Behaviour Change* (3rd edn). New York: John Wiley.

GOLDBERG, D. P., HOBSON, R. F., MAGUIRE, G. P. *et al* (1984) The clarification and assessment of a method of psychotherapy. *British Journal of Psychiatry*, **144**, 567–575.

GOMES-SCHWARTZ, B. (1982) Negative change induced by psychotherapy. *British Journal of Hospital Medicine*, **28**, 248–253.

GORDON, W. A., FRIEDENBERGS, I., DILLER, L. *et al* (1980) Efficacy of psychosocial intervention with cancer patients. *Journal of Consulting and Clinical Psychology*, **48**, 743–759.

GOTTMAN, J. & MARKMAN, H. J. (1978) Experimental designs in psychotherapy research. In *Handbook of Psychotherapy and Behaviour Change* (2nd edn) (eds S. L. Garfield & A. E. Bergin), pp. 23–62. New York: John Wiley.

HERINK, R. (ed.) (1980) *The Psychotherapy Handbook*. New York: New American Library.

HOBSON, R. F. (1985) *Forms of Feeling: The Heart of Psychotherapy*. London: Tavistock.

KAGAN, N. (1980) Eighteen years with IPR. In *Psychotherapy Supervision: Theory, Research and Practice* (ed. A. K. Hess). London: John Wiley.

KANDEL, H. J., AYLLON, T. & ROSENBAUM, M. S. (1977) Flooding or systematic exposure in the treatment of extreme social withdrawal in children. *Journal of Behaviour Therapy and Experimental Psychiatry*, **8**, 75–81.

KAZDIN, A. E. (1986) The evaluation of psychotherapy: research design and methodology. In *Handbook of Psychotherapy and Behaviour Change* (3rd edn) (eds S. L. Garfield & A. E. Bergin), pp. 23–60. New York: John Wiley.

—— & WILCOXON, L. (1976) Systematic desensitization and non-specific treatment effects. *Psychological Bulletin*, **83**, 729–758.

KRASNER, L. (1962) The therapist as social reinforcement machine. In *Research in Psychotherapy*, vol. II (eds H. H. Strupp & L. Luborsky). Washington, DC: American Psychological Association.

LAMBERT, M. J., CHRISTENSEN, E. R. & DE JULIO, S. S. (1983) *The Assessment of Psychotherapy Outcome*. New York: Wiley-Interscience.

LANCET (1984) Editorial – Psychotherapy: effective treatment or expensive placebo? *Lancet*, i, 83–84.

LUBORSKY, L., SINGER, B. & LUBORSKY, L. (1975) Comparative studies of the psycho- therapies: is it true that "everyone has won and all must have prizes"? *Archives of General Psychiatry*, **32**, 995–1008.

MAGUIRE, P., TAIT, A., BROOKE, M. *et al* (1980) Effect of counselling on the psychiatric morbidity associated with mastectomy. *British Medical Journal*, **281**, 1454–1456.

MAGUIRE, G. P., GOLDBERG, D. P., HOBSON, R. F., *et al* (1984) Evaluating the teaching of a method of psychotherapy. *British Journal of Psychiatry*, **144**, 575–580.

MALAN, D. H., SHELDON HEATH, E., BACAL, H. A., *et al* (1975) Psychodynamic changes in untreated patients II: apparently genuine improvements. *Archives of General Psychiatry*, **32**, 110–126.

MARGISON, F. & HOBSON, R. F. (1983) *A Conversational Model of Psychotherapy: A Videotape Teaching Package*. London: Tavistock.

MCGRATH, G. & LOWSON, K. (1987) Assessing the benefits of psychotherapy: the economic approach. *British Journal of Psychiatry*, **150**, 65–71.

MULHALL, D. (1976) Systematic self-assessment by PQRST. *Psychological Medicine*, **6**, 591–597.

ORLINSKY, D. E. & HOWARD, K. I. (1986) The psychological interior of psychotherapy: explorations with the therapy session reports. In *The Psychotherapeutic Process: A Research Handbook* (eds L. S. Greenberg & W. M. Pinsoff). New York: Guildford Press.

PAUL, G. L. (1966) *Insight versus Desensitisation in Psychotherapy: An Experiment in Anxiety Reduction*. Stanford: Stanford University Press.

PECK, D. F. (1985) Small N designs in clinical research. In *New Developments in Clinical Psychology* (ed. F. Watts). London: John Wiley.

PLUM, A. (1981) Communication as skill: a critique and alternative proposal. *Journal of Humanistic Psychology*, **21**, 3–19.

ROSSER, R., DENFORD, J., HESLOP, A., *et al* (1983) Breathlessness and psychiatric morbidity in chronic bronchitis and emphysema: a study of psychotherapeutic management. *Psychological Medicine*, **13**, 93–110.

SHAPIRO, A. K. (1984) Opening comments: "What works with what?". Psychotherapy efficacy for specific disorders – an overview of the research. In *Psychotherapy Research; Where Are We and Where Should We Go?* (eds J. B. Williams & R. L. Spitzer) New York: Guildford.

—— & HOBSON, R. F. (1972) Preliminary communication: change in psychotherapy – a single case study. *Psychological Medicine*, **2**, 312–317.

——, & SHAPIRO, D. (1982) Meta analysis of comparative therapy outcome studies: a replication and refinement. *Psychological Bulletin*, **92**, 581–604.

—— & —— (1983) Comparative therapy outcome research: methodological implications of meta-analysis. *Journal of Consulting and Clinical Psychology*, **51**, 42–53.

—— & FIRTH, J. (1987) Prescriptive v. exploratory psychotherapy: outcomes of the Sheffield psychotherapy project. *British Journal of Psychiatry*, **151**, 790–799.

SHEPHERD, M. (1984) Editorial – What price psychotherapy? *British Medical Journal*, **288**, 809–810.

SMITH, M. L. & GLASS, G. V. (1977) Meta-analysis of psychotherapy outcome studies. *American Psychologist*, **32**, 752–760.

STERN, R. & MARKS, I. M. (1973) Brief and prolonged flooding. *Archives of General Psychiatry*, **28**, 270–276.

STILES, W. B. (1979) Verbal response mode and psychotherapeutic technique. *Psychiatry*, **42**, 49–62.

——, SHAPIRO, D. A. & ELLIOTT, R. (1986) Are all psychotherapies equivalent? *American Psychologist*, **41**, 165–180.

STORR, A. (1979) *The Art of Psychotherapy*. London: William Heinemann.

WASKOW, I. E. (1984) Specification of the technique variable in the NIMH Treatment of Depression Collaborative Research Program. In *Psychotherapy Research* (eds J. B. W. Williams & R. L. Spitzer). London: Guildford Press.

—— & PARLOFF, M. B. (1975) *Psychotherapy Change Measures*. Washington, D.C: DHEW.

WEISSMAN, M. M. (1979) The psychological treatment of depression: evidence for the efficacy of psychotherapy alone, in comparison with, and in combination with pharmacotherapy. *Archives of General Psychiatry*, **36**, 1261–1269.

——, PRUSOFF, B. A., DIMASCIO, A., *et al* (1979) The efficacy of drugs and psychotherapy in the treatment of acute depressive episodes. *American Journal of Psychiatry*, **136**, 555–558.

WILKINSON, G. (1984) Editorial – psychotherapy in the market place. *Psychological Medicine*, **14**, 23–26.

7 Long-term outcome studies of psychological treatments

KEITH HAWTON

Research into psychological treatments has largely been concerned with the immediate effects of treatment and the extent to which therapeutic gains are sustained in the short term. Relatively little attention has been paid to the longer-term outcome. There are several reasons for this (Table 7.1), including the practical difficulties inherent in organising long-term outcome studies, the complex issues which bedevil interpretation of their results, and the fact that most treatment research is funded on a relatively short-term basis, which does not allow for longer-term assessment of outcome. Furthermore, some of the disinclination towards long-term outcome studies may be the result of previous investigators (e.g. Stone *et al* 1961; Paul, 1967) having declared that evaluation of psychological treatments should be primarily in terms of immediate results. While there is no doubt that controlled evaluation of treatment is easier to maintain in the short term, it is important also to consider longer-term outcome.

This chapter, in addition to reviewing the reasons why long-term outcome studies are important, examines the design of such studies, the difficulties they pose, and how these can be reduced. While there is no clear distinction between the short term and the long term, and indeed one can argue that this might differ according to the type of disorder and condition being studied, an arbitrary time of one year or more following treatment has been adopted to distinguish long-term from short-term outcome.

Importance of long-term outcome studies

Long-term outcome studies of patients who have received psychological treatments are important because they can:

(a) demonstrate persistent effects of treatment
(b) examine the preventive effects of treatment

TABLE 7.1
Comparison of short-term and long-term treatment studies

	Short term	Long term
Feasibility	Good	Poor or difficult to predict
Cost	Relatively cheap	Expensive if comprehensive
Ethics	Few problems if period of treatment is short	Ethical doubts if treatment is restricted over a long period
Quality of data	Assured if personnel are constant and well trained	Variable standard because of changes in instruments, attitudes and personnel
Tracing rate	High	Low

(c) identify the problems patients encounter following treatment
(d) identify predictors of outcome
(e) examine patients' long-term attitudes to treatment
(f) detect any iatrogenic consequences of treatment.

Persistence of treatment effects

It could be argued that it is difficult to justify time-consuming therapy if it can be shown to produce only short-term benefits, unless this is on the grounds that amelioration of immediate distress is a justified objective (even if this effect is short lived). Thus the most obvious reason for conducting long-term outcome studies is to assess whether or not therapeutic effects persist. One reason for the disappearance of a short-term difference between patients who received an experimental treatment and those who were in a control group is that the effects of the experimental treatment do not persist; another is that spontaneous improvement among patients in the control group can negate the original differences between the groups.

The greatest impact of psychological treatments is usually immediate. However, this is not always the case, treatment effects sometimes being expected to manifest themselves more clearly a while after treatment has ended. Individual psychotherapy and marital therapy are two examples. Assessment of long-term outcome is then essential in order to determine whether the predicted effect actually occurs.

Long-term follow-up studies can also identify particular subgroups of patients who have a different outcome compared with the rest of a sample, in spite of their immediate outcomes having been similar. Such a finding can demonstrate the necessity of trying out different approaches with such subgroups in order to try to produce a more sustained effect. An example of this is provided by two recent long-term outcome studies of couples who had entered sex therapy between one and six years earlier. While the effects of treatment were reasonably sustained in many patients, couples who had originally presented because of the female partner's impaired interest in sex often had an extremely poor long-term outcome, in spite of the initial outcome having been only a little inferior to that of couples with other sexual dysfunctions (De Amicis *et al*, 1985; Hawton *et al*, 1986). These studies have emphasised the need to reappraise current treatment approaches and devise novel methods of therapy for couples presenting with this problem.

The preventive effects of treatment

Prevention of further episodes of illness will usually be a major objective of treatment for episodic psychiatric disorders. Long-term follow-up is then imperative in order to determine whether this objective is fulfilled.

Examples are provided by studies which have evaluated treatment intended to modify the interactions between schizophrenic patients and their relatives. One study identified patients at special risk of relapse because of their extensive social contact with relatives who were frequently critical of them (high 'expressed emotion'). Half of the patients received intensive psychosocial intervention aimed at altering the nature and extent of interaction between themselves and their relatives, while the other half received traditional care. Patients in a second study were also at high risk of relapse because they lived in stressful home environments. Half received family intervention, which was intended to improve the problem-solving capacity of the patients and their relatives, and the other half traditional care. Two-year follow-up in both studies revealed far fewer relapses in the experimental groups than in controls (Leff *et al*, 1985; Falloon *et al*, 1985). While these results must be interpreted with some caution because other factors might have explained the results (e.g. better compliance with medication in the experimental groups), they do provide encouraging support for psychosocial approaches (combined with medication) to the care of patients with schizophrenia.

Research into cognitive therapy for depression provides another example. Proponents of cognitive therapy have suggested that not only may it be at least as effective as antidepressant treatment in the short term, but it is also likely to reduce the risk of further episodes of depression. This is because in the course of treatment patients are taught that affective symptoms relate to patterns of thinking which can be modified by their own efforts, and considerable attention is also paid to identifying and altering underlying dysfunctional attitudes that may be a source of distorted thinking (Beck *et al*, 1979). This suggested effect on future risk of depression has now received support from two follow-up studies, the first of outcome a year after treatment (Simons *et al*, 1986) and the second two years after treatment (Blackburn *et al*, 1986), both of which demonstrated a reduced number of subsequent episodes of depression in patients who received cognitive therapy, either alone or in combination with drug treatment, compared with those who received only drug treatment, even among patients who had responded equally well to the initial treatment. A third study found no difference in outcome one year after treatment between patients who had received cognitive therapy and those who had received imipramine, although there had been better immediate symptomatic improvement and a higher treatment completion rate in those in the psychologically treated group (Kovacs *et al*, 1981).

Further support for the longer-term benefits of psychological treatment compared with antidepressants has been provided by Weissman *et al* (1981). They demonstrated that while nearly all the depressed patients who had entered a trial comparing brief focal interpersonal psychotherapy with antidepressant treatment and with combined treatment had a good outcome one year later, patients who had received interpersonal psychotherapy, with or without the antidepressant, showed better social adjustment than those who had received the antidepressant only.

Anticipation of problems following treatment

Long-term follow-up studies can also provide information about the types of difficulties patients commonly experience following treatment and possible methods of coping with these. With this knowledge a therapist is in a much better position to advise future patients what problems they may face and how they might prepare for them. Studies of phobic patients have shown, for example, that reappearance of a phobia, albeit often temporarily, is not uncommon in the face of adverse life events (e.g. Burns *et al*, 1986). A follow-up investigation of couples who had entered sex therapy between one and six years previously demonstrated that they commonly experienced further sexual difficulties, that these were often temporary, and that communication between the partners, practising the approaches learned during therapy, and adopting an accepting approach to the difficulty, appeared to be the most effective means of coping (Hawton *et al*, 1986).

Predictors of outcome

Long-term outcome studies can also allow early predictors of eventual outcome to be identified. Such information may not only be important in allowing more informed decisions to be made about whether or not treatment should be continued in refractory cases, but can also alert therapists to patients who may need especially intensive or prolonged therapy. Thus one follow-up study of depressed patients, most of whom had received cognitive therapy, showed that the level of dysfunctional attitudes and of depression at the end of treatment were significant predictors of subsequent relapse or remission (Simons *et al*, 1986). Follow-up of patients with obsessive–compulsive disorders whose treatment had consisted of exposure and response prevention, while demonstrating excellent outcome for most subjects, especially in terms of their compulsions, also showed that patients who were convinced of the realistic nature of their fears were likely to have a poor outcome (Foa & Goldstein, 1978).

Attitudes to treatment

Differences may be found in patients' attitudes to therapy and to specific components of a treatment programme, depending on whether they are assessed immediately after treatment has been completed, when a halo effect might be operating, or much later. Ideally, attitudes should be assessed in both the short and long term. One example of a study in which attitudes to treatment were investigated at long-term follow-up has been reported by Burns *et al* (1986), who assessed patients eight years after they had received behaviour therapy for agoraphobia. They cited the following as the most important components of therapy: exposure *in vivo*; being pushed to go out more, or getting into a routine of going out; relaxation training; encouragement, reassurance, and sympathy from the therapist; and the use of coping skills or self-instructions. Similarly, in a follow-up study of couples who had entered sex therapy, the partners reported that the most helpful ingredients of treatment had been the homework assignments (in terms of their impact on communication between the partners and their awareness of each other), attention to improving their understanding of their problem, and stress reduction (Hawton *et al*, 1986). Information such as this can be used to ensure that subsequent treatment programmes emphasise these components.

Iatrogenic effects of treatment

An often cited criticism of behaviour therapy, particularly by its early critics, was that it was likely to result in 'symptom substitution' (the replacement of an earlier symptom by a different one) because it did not tackle the fundamental or intrapsychic causes of psychological problems. This and other allegations that a treatment can create new (iatrogenic) problems can be tested only by long-term follow-up of treated patients. Several follow-up studies of phobic patients treated by behavioural methods have now convincingly demonstrated that successfully treated patients rarely develop a new symptom or disorder (Paul, 1967; Marks, 1971; Emmelkamp & Kuipers, 1979; McPherson *et al*, 1980; Munby & Johnston, 1980).

Design of long-term outcome studies

The different designs used in long-term outcome studies are summarised in Table 7.2. They differ in the extent to which treatment is controlled and the nature of the populations used for comparison.

Follow-up of patients who have all entered one type of treatment

Several long-term follow-up studies have included only patients who have received, or at least entered, one type of treatment. A major drawback of

TABLE 7.2
Experimental designs in long-term treatment studies

Design	Advantages	Disadvantages
Parallel design of treated/ untreated populations	Comparison groups ideal when available	'Untreated' groups are usually contaminated by some treatment
Comparison of cohort with historical equivalent	Previous data already available	Past data include too many uncontrolled variables
Variation in timing of treatment (waiting-list control)	Easy to effect as it is often close to normal clinical practice	Differences in outcome tend to disappear in the long term
Simple follow-up with no control group (naturalistic study)	No ethical problems as additional treatments are allowed	Impossible to separate natural history of disorder from effects of treatment

such studies is the difficulty of attributing changes found during the follow-up period, or at the follow-up assessment, to the effects of treatment itself. Possible methods of evaluating treatment effects include the following.

(a) The outcome of treated patients can be compared with findings for untreated samples of patients with the same disorder. The latter can provide information on the extent to which patients improve without treatment ('spontaneous remission'). However, data on untreated samples of patients similar to those who receive treatment are rarely available. One example was reported by Agras *et al* (1972), who showed that untreated adult phobics improved very little over a five-year period. Another was provided by Segraves *et al* (1982), who found a 15% spontaneous remission rate among men with psychogenic erectile dysfunction who had been assessed in a psychiatric clinic one year earlier, a figure much lower than that found in treatment outcome studies.

(b) Another approach is to compare the outcome of treated patients with that of comparable patients treated by different methods in the past. However, inadequacy of previous outcome measures is usually a severe limitation.

(c) Use of a protracted baseline or waiting period before patients enter treatment can provide some sort of control against which later changes can be compared. One example of this was a study of controlled breathing as a treatment for patients with a panic complaint, in which a stable baseline was established before treatment (Clark *et al*, 1985). Because the substantial improvements with treatment occurred in a shorter time than the baseline period, it seemed reasonable to accept the changes as treatment effects. Maintenance of these gains persisted at two-year follow-up (although additional treatment had usually been provided). While baseline measures can never provide fully adequate comparison, changes following an experimental treatment can more reliably be attributed to the treatment itself if the waiting period has been relatively long.

Despite the considerable problem of identifying treatment effects, uncontrolled follow-up studies can generate much useful information, especially with regard to the types of further difficulties patients face after treatment, effective means of coping with these, predictors of outcome, patients' attitudes to treatment, possible symptom substitution and factors associated with relapse. Research workers therefore should certainly not be discouraged from conducting this type of follow-up study; it can often be surprisingly informative.

Follow-up of patients who have entered controlled treatment studies

The type of follow-up study that would provide the most useful information would be one in which patients had originally been randomly assigned to either an experimental treatment group or a control group. The latter would have received either no treatment, or a conventional or comparison treatment. No further therapy would have been provided during a lengthy follow-up period, at the end of which the two groups would be compared. Unfortunately, such a study is impractical, for at least two reasons. First, it is usually unethical to withhold treatment from patients for more than a brief period. Second, patients in a less effective treatment group are likely to have received further help during the follow-up period, either from the original treatment agency or from other sources.

These factors, which are clearly likely to reduce the *apparent* effectiveness of an otherwise more effective experimental treatment, are nicely illustrated by a thorough follow-up study of agoraphobic patients who had all received some form of treatment during one of three controlled treatment studies of behaviour therapy between five and nine years earlier (Munby & Johnston, 1980). Six patients in the first treatment study had received non-behavioural therapy ('associative psychotherapy') that had proved ineffective at the time (Gelder *et al*, 1973). At follow-up these patients were indistinguishable from those treated by behavioural methods. However, since the end of the original treatment, three had received behaviour therapy, one had been treated intensively as an in-patient, and one had undergone psychosurgery.

One means of taking account of 'hidden' differences in long-term effectiveness between treatments is to compare the extent to which further treatment (psychological and pharmacological) has been sought or received since the end of the original treatment. If it can be clearly demonstrated that patients who originally received treatment X have had significantly less treatment during the follow-up period than patients who received treatment Y, this supports a claim for the greater efficacy of X compared with Y. However, one potential criticism of this method of evaluation is that it relies to a large extent on the help-seeking behaviour of patients, which itself may have been influenced by the original treatment. For example, it is possible that patients who receive cognitive therapy for depression do *not* have fewer episodes of depression subsequently than patients who receive drug treatment, but because of the nature of the original treatment become more able to tolerate further symptoms and/or more reluctant to seek help (Blackburn *et al*, 1986). This effect, while perhaps unlikely, is nevertheless a possibility with 'naturalistic' follow-up studies (see below).

Methods used in long-term outcome studies

There are basically two types of follow-up study, 'controlled' and 'naturalistic'. In the former, patients remain in specific treatment groups throughout the follow-up period, and do not receive any different type of treatment. As already noted, it is virtually impossible to conduct this type of study entirely successfully if the follow-up period is to be protracted, especially if the original condition for which treatment was offered was at all serious. In naturalistic studies, once treatment has been completed there are no restraints on whatever type of further help patients might seek or receive. Most follow-up studies are of this kind.

Three means of assessment may be employed in follow-up studies: interview, postal questionnaire, and indirect measures.

Interview

Face-to-face interviews with patients are usually the most valuable method of follow-up, especially for assessing specific problems and symptoms, and investigating whether further difficulties have been experienced since treatment ended and how these were managed. Assessment measures might include specific assessment of the original problem for which help was sought, mood questionnaires to assess general symptoms and a specially designed structured interview to obtain information about, for example, further episodes of difficulty since treatment ended, how these were managed, and attitudes to the original treatment. The long-term outcome study reported by Munby & Johnston (1980) of patients who had received treatment for agoraphobia provides a good example of a reasonably comprehensive evaluation at follow-up. Thus patients were assessed with regard to: (a) agoraphobia, by means of two self-rated scales – an assessor's rating and diaries concerning time recently spent out of the house (these were only completed by a subgroup of patients who had also completed them in relation to the original treatment); (b) anxiety and depression, by the assessor's ratings and a self-rated mood scale; and (c) further treatment received, by means of a structured questionnaire.

Serial measures can be obtained if interviews are conducted at regular intervals. However, this is labour intensive and expensive. Most long-term follow-up studies therefore rely on a single interview. While allowing satisfactory assessment of current symptoms and problems, this means that further episodes of disorder since treatment ended but before the follow-up must be identified by retrospective inquiry either about symptoms, which can be unreliable, or about further help received or sought. The value of interviews can be increased if information can also be obtained from another informant, such as a relative.

Postal questionnaires

For economic and practical reasons some follow-up studies are based on postal questionnaires sent to patients, rather than face-to-face interview. This can have the advantage of increasing the 'catch rate', especially of patients who may have moved away. However, information obtained by postal questionnaire is less reliable and usually less extensive than that obtained at interview.

Indirect measures

Studies which rely on indirect measures of progress collect information only from sources other than patients themselves, such as from medical and other official records. This type of investigation will obviously be restricted to the identification of factors such as major episodes of illness, prescribing of medication, and behaviour (e.g. suicide attempts) which might be detected through official records. In countries such as Sweden, where extensive official records are maintained on the whole population, this type of study can be particularly productive. Ettlinger (1975), for example, used this approach in Sweden to conduct a five-year follow-up investigation of two groups of attempted suicide patients, one of which had been offered a special after-care service and the other traditional care. Official records allowed completed suicide, repeat attempts, and a crude measure of social functioning to be used as outcome variables. However, the range of information provided by this type of follow-up study will always be limited.

Follow-up studies often utilise a combination of the above approaches, with for example, interviews with patients, postal questionnaire inquiry of patients not available for interview, and scrutiny of general practice or hospital records. Telephone interviews are often used to overcome geographical limitations and are particularly popular in the United States.

Difficulties encountered in long-term outcome studies

It will by now be clear to the reader that this type of investigation is far from easy. While most of the commonly encountered difficulties have already been mentioned, three are of special concern, and these are discussed below.

Loss of cases at follow-up

Long-term outcome studies frequently suffer from loss of subjects. This may be for a variety of reasons, including refusal to be seen, mobility, inability to trace, and death. The most serious problem here is not necessarily the actual number of subjects contacted, but the extent to which these are representative of the original group. Some of the reasons for loss of subjects are also likely to mean that those who can be followed up are atypical, both in terms of their outcome at the end of treatment (treatment failures often being more difficult to follow-up) and other characteristics (e.g. compliance) which may be relevant to eventual outcome.

Investigators should do all they can to maximise follow-up rates. It is helpful to plan follow-up studies well in advance, preferably when the original treatment phase is designed, because patients can be told at the outset that they will be contacted again well after the end of treatment. This may increase compliance. Obtaining extensive information about how contact might be made at follow-up should the person have moved house (e.g. having the telephone number of a relative who is likely to know of the patient's new address) can also help.

In spite of the researcher's best efforts, loss of subjects is likely to occur. A separate analysis should always be carried out for comparability of the followed up sample with those patients lost to follow-up. In addition to demographic characteristics, such comparison should include severity of the presenting problem and other symptoms before the original treatment, initial response to the treatment, and any other factors likely to be important in determining eventual outcome. Matching of the followed up sample with the original sample can sometimes be achieved by omitting from analysis cases that make the followed up sample atypical. However, since this will often result in reduction of the sample to an unacceptable size, the only option may be to report the results in a way that makes absolutely clear any atypical features of the sample and the likely effect of these in terms of the estimated outcome of the whole group.

How to define further episodes of disorder

The critical dependent variable in much long-term outcome research is the extent to which there have been further episodes of the disorder for which treatment was originally provided. A particular difficulty is knowing whether the symptoms represent reappearance of the original episode or a new episode of illness. This becomes even more difficult when recovery from the original episode was incomplete, or was defined as a fall in symptom score below a certain level on a questionnaire.

The terms 'relapse' and 'recurrence' are used to indicate reappearance of symptoms after symptom-free periods. 'Relapse' is typically used to denote recurrence of the initial episode and is therefore applied if symptoms reappear after a short time, and 'recurrence' for a new episode, when symptoms recur after a longer period of time. Klerman (1978) has attempted to make these vague concepts more definite by applying arbitrary criteria, namely that relapse should be used for return of symptoms within six to nine months of the onset of the original episode, and recurrence for return of symptoms after that period.

However, while this simple classification may help, it leaves a more serious difficulty, namely *what* constitutes return of symptoms or disorder. To illustrate this in the case of depression, criteria which might be used include exceeding a cut-off score on a questionnaire such as the Beck Depression Inventory; development of symptoms to an extent that they meet the criteria for major depression; and re-referral to treatment for depression. All of these criteria have potential drawbacks, the first two (especially the first) because they may overestimate recurrence (type I error) and the last because it may underestimate recurrence (type II error). Similar but even more complex problems are encountered in defining recurrence of schizophrenia (Falloon *et al*, 1983).

These issues should be addressed in follow-up studies, and either more than one type of criterion used, or else one that represents the best compromise.

Effects of uncontrollable events

A follow-up period, however short, can never be a vacuum in which there are no influences other than the original treatment. A study of the effects of life events on outcome in a trial comparing three types of psychotherapy (individual, group, and conjoint) did not reveal a significant effect during a seven-month follow-up (Pilkonis *et al*, 1984). However, when a follow-up is lengthy, major life events and difficulties are likely to have a major impact on a patient's psychological status and therefore to affect potential differences between treatment groups. To exemplify this in extreme form, if two patients had been equally successfully treated for depression, but during the follow-up period one had experienced the death of a spouse and the other had had no troubles, it would hardly be surprising if the second appeared to have a better long-term outcome. Therefore in some outcome studies the extent to which life events and difficulties have occurred since the end of treatment has been measured, using one of the available life-event interviews or questionnaires. In doing this it is essential to distinguish life events and difficulties that are the result of recurrence or persistence of psychiatric disorder and those that are clearly independent of any disorder. However, it remains unclear how best to control for such stresses, especially if they are not evenly distributed between groups of patients. One approach is to omit all subjects who have experienced very major independent stresses; another is to omit cases sufficient to allow balancing across treatment groups. Neither solution is entirely satisfactory.

Conclusions

Despite the many difficulties encountered when studying longer-term outcome following psychological treatment, this type of investigation is extremely important. Indeed, it can be argued that satisfaction concerning the apparent benefits of a treatment method is fully valid only if such benefits can be shown to persist to at least some degree in the longer term. Furthermore, evaluation of some forms of treatment, especially those concerned with prevention of relapse, must rely on assessment of long-term outcome.

Regrettably, the design of long-term outcome studies is generally inferior to that for short-term outcome. Researchers should take account of the desirability of assessing outcome in the long term when initially designing treatment studies. While some of the limitations of long-term outcome studies may be unavoidable, careful design can reduce these and hence maximise the usefulness of information which can be obtained.

Recommended reading

Helpful discussions of the methodology and difficulties of long-term follow-up studies are given by Paul (1967) and Blackburn *et al* (1986), and of the problems of defining recurrence of illness by Klerman (1978) and Falloon *et al* (1983). Specific reports of long-term follow-up studies which the reader might find useful when planning their own research include Paul (1967), Munby & Johnston (1980), Weissman *et al* (1981), Blackburn *et al* (1986) and Hawton *et al* (1986).

References

AGRAS, W. S., CHAPIN, H. W., JACKSON, M., *et al* (1972) The natural history of phobia. *Archives of General Psychiatry*, **26**, 315–317.

BLACKBURN, I. M., EUNSON, K. M. & BISHOP, S. (1986) A two-year naturalistic follow-up of depressed patients treated with cognitive therapy, pharmacotherapy and a combination of both. *Journal of Affective Disorders*, **10**, 67–75.

BECK, A. T., RUSH, A. J., SHAW, B. F., *et al* (1979) *Cognitive Therapy of Depression*. New York: Guildford Press.

BURNS, L. E., THORPE, G. L. & CAVALLARO, L. A. (1986) Agoraphobia 8 years after behavioural treatment: a follow-up study with interview, self-report, and behavioural data. *Behavior Therapy*, **17**, 580–591.

CLARK, D. M., SALKOVSKIS, P. M. & CHALKLEY, A. J. (1985) Respiratory control as a treatment for panic attacks. *Journal of Behavior Therapy and Experimental Psychiatry*, **16**, 23–30.

DE AMICIS, L. A., GOLDBERG, D. C., LoPICCOLO, J., *et al* (1985) Clinical follow-up of couples treated for sexual dysfunction. *Archives of Sexual Behavior*, **14**, 467–489.

EMMELKAMP, P. M. G. & KUIPERS, A. C. M. (1979) Agoraphobia: a follow-up study four years after treatment. *British Journal of Psychiatry*, **134**, 352–355.

ETTLINGER, R. (1975) Evaluation of suicide prevention after attempted suicide. *Acta Psychiatrica Scandinavica* (suppl. 260).

FALLOON, I. R. H., MARSHALL, G. N., BOYD, J. L., *et al* (1983) Relapse in schizophrenia: a review of the concept and its definitions. *Psychological Medicine*, **13**, 469–477.

——, BOYD, L. F., McGILL, C. W., *et al* (1985) Family management in the prevention of morbidity of schizophrenia: clinical outcome of a two-year longitudinal study. *Archives of General Psychiatry*, **42**, 887–896.

FOA, E. B. & GOLDSTEIN, A. (1978) Continuous exposure and complete response prevention in the treatment of obsessive–compulsive neurosis. *Behavior Therapy*, **9**, 821–829.

GELDER, M. G., BANCROFT, J. H. J., GATH, D. H., *et al* (1973) Specific and non-specific factors in behaviour therapy. *British Journal of Psychiatry*, **123**, 445–462.

HAWTON, K., CATALAN, J., MARTIN, P., *et al* (1986) Long-term outcome of sex therapy. *Behaviour Research and Therapy*, **24**, 665–675.

KLERMAN, G. L. (1978) Long-term maintenance of affective disorders. In *Psychopharmacology: A Generation of Progress* (eds M. A. Lipton, A. Dimascio & K. Killam), pp. 1302–1311. New York: Raven Press.

KOVACS, M., RUSH, A. J., BECK, A. T., *et al* (1981) Depressed outpatients treated with cognitive therapy or pharmacotherapy: one year follow-up. *Archives of General Psychiatry*, **38**, 33–39.

LEFF, J., KUIPERS, L., BERKOWITZ, R., *et al* (1985) A controlled trial of social intervention in the families of schizophrenic patients: two year follow-up. *British Journal of Psychiatry*, **146**, 594–600.

MARKS, I. (1971) Phobic disorders four years after treatment: a prospective follow-up. *British Journal of Psychiatry*, **118**, 683–688.

McPHERSON, F. M., BROUGHAM, L. & McLAREN, S. (1980) Maintenance of improvement in agoraphobic patients treated by behavioural methods – a four year follow-up. *Behaviour Research and Behaviour*, **18**, 150–152.

MUNBY, M. & JOHNSTON, D. W. (1980) Agoraphobia: the long-term follow-up of behavioural treatment. *British Journal of Psychiatry*, **137**, 418–427.

PAUL, G. L. (1967) Insight versus desensitization in psychotherapy two years after termination. *Journal of Consulting Psychology*, **31**, 333–348.

PILKONIS, P. A., IMBER, S. D. & RUBINSKY, P. (1984) Influence of life events on outcome in psychotherapy. *Journal of Nervous and Mental Disease*, **172**, 468–474.

SEGRAVES, R. T., KNOPF, J. & CAMIC, P. (1982) Spontaneous remission in erectile impotence. *Behavioural Research and Therapy*, **20**, 89–91.

SIMONS, A. D., MURPHY, G. E., LEVINE, J. L., *et al* (1986) Cognitive therapy and pharmacotherapy for depression. *Archives of General Psychiatry*, **43**, 43–48.

STONE, A. R., FRANK, J. D., NASH, E. H., *et al* (1961) An intensive five-year follow-up study of treated psychiatric outpatients. *Journal of Nervous and Mental Disease*, **133**, 410–422.

WEISSMAN, M. M., KLERMAN, G. L., PRUSOFF, B. A., *et al* (1981) Depressed outpatients: results one year after treatment with drugs and/or interpersonal psychotherapy. *Archives of General Psychiatry*, **38**, 51–55.

8 Principles of psychological assessment

STEPHEN MORLEY and PHILIP SNAITH

The aims of this chapter are threefold: to provide the reader with an introduction to basic issues that surround measurement of psychological and behavioural variables; to provide a series of guidelines which potential researchers may use when setting up projects (throughout this chapter the reader will find check-lists which summarise major points); and to provide a useful bibliography.

Current research in psychiatry covers a very wide range of problems and raises a spectrum of measurement problems such as case detection, assessing the severity of a disorder, and assessing personality, mood, intellectual performance and behavioural activity. Measures may be required to categorise people on salient dimensions or to index change during therapeutic trials. To meet these demands a series of techniques is used, ranging across observer rating scales for interviews, behavioural observation studies, self-rating scales for personality and mood measurement, and self-monitoring methods (usually 'diaries') used in therapeutic trials. Measures may have group-referenced norms which enable a person to be located with respect to a defined target population, or, at the other extreme, personal questionnaire techniques which provide sensitive measurement tailored to one person may be used. Given this range of measurement problems and methods, is it possible to provide a framework by which the researcher can evaluate his/her requirements, select an appropriate measure and interpret the results which arise from his/her investigation?

The concepts of validity and reliability, developed by psychometricians, do provide such an evaluative framework and they have great utility; this chapter provides an overview of them and shows that they are not separate concepts but are closely intertwined and can be placed within a relatively new notion of generalisability which has so far not penetrated psychiatric research.

Validity

On beginning research one is often asked to state whether a selected measure is reliable and valid. Generally this question is misleading because it implies that there are single indices of reliability (discussed under a separate heading, below) and validity, and that the measure is reliable and valid for all occasions on which it is used. It is also implied that a test has *inherent* validity. This is strictly not true; what is validated is an interpretation of data obtained by the test under specified conditions, and a test which has validity under one set of measurement conditions may not be valid when applied to another problem in another context, although the situation may be superficially similar.

Content validity

Content validity is concerned with whether the instrument adequately probes the specific domain that one requires. For example a test of mathematical reasoning would have no content validity as a measure of verbal ability (although it may have considerable predictive validity and construct validity – see below). Content validity is a serious problem in psychiatry, especially

TABLE 8.1

A comparison of the contents of two scales for measuring depression, the BDI and the depression subscale of the HAD scale

BDI	HAD
Items shared by the BDI and HAD	
Pessimism	Current enjoyment
Current dissatisfaction	Current laughter
Sad feeling	Feel cheerful
Feel unattractive	Loss of interest in appearance
Discouraged about future	Anticipated enjoyment
	(a) general
	(b) from books and TV
Effort to work	Slowed down
BDI items not in the HAD	
Past failure	
Punishment	
Self-blame	
Crying	
Loss of interest in others	
Guilt	
Disappointed in self	
Self-harm	
Irritable	
Decision difficulties	
*Sleep	
*Appetite	
*Weight loss	
*Concern with health	
*Libido	

While both scales contain items that refer to anhedonic state, the BDI contains many additional items. The items marked with an asterisk might be checked by patients with physical illness because they are physically ill rather than depressed.

when in diagnosis one must consider the selection of appropriate symptoms, the required level of severity of the symptoms and the time frame in which these symptoms are to be measured (Williams *et al*, 1980). A scale will have content validity insofar as it does not contain elements that could be attributable to other processes, or variables that are not the focus of the disorder to be studied. In order to establish content validity, investigators must have clearly articulated 'maps' of what they want to measure.

Example: measuring depression in physical illness

The problem here is that the traditional psychiatric concept of depression includes the presence of 'biological symptoms' such as loss of appetite and sleep disturbance. These symptoms are often present in physical illness although the person may not be depressed. It is therefore necessary to map a revised concept of depression in this group of people and to develop a measuring instrument which taps the revised map and is therefore uncontaminated by symptoms that can arise primarily through ill health and are not attributable to depression. Zigmond & Snaith (1983) report the development of such an instrument, the Hospital Anxiety and Depression (HAD) scale, and Table 8.1 illustrates the relationship of the concept of depression as assessed by the depression subscale of the HAD compared with that of the widely used Beck Depression Inventory (BDI; Beck *et al*, 1961).

Arguments about the content validity of instruments are therefore concerned with the specification of theories about what one is trying to measure. There are no empirical methods of justifying content validity – one cannot refer to correlations between the test and other measures as an index of content validity. Content validity is obtained only by developing a conceptual map of what one wants to measure and considering what other factors would contaminate the measure. The important step in preparing a research project is therefore to define carefully the variable one wishes to measure and the populations and conditions under which the measurement is to take place. Potential measuring instruments can then be inspected for their content and the way in which it was derived. One then chooses the 'best-fit' measure. In some cases it may be necessary to tailor the instrument to one's own needs or develop a new measure.

Checklist for content validity

▷ Specify carefully what you want to measure.
▷ Inspect measures already available.
    How well do their contents match what you want to measure?
    How were the contents of these instruments derived?
    Does this match your requirements?

Criterion validity

Criterion validity determines whether a measure discriminates between people who are known to be dissimilar on a feature external to the measure itself. Many measures are developed as a cost-effective way of classifying people without the need for extensive interviews by clinicians. The criterion validity of these tests is therefore very important and their development will include calibration against reliable external criteria. The General Health Questionnaire (GHQ; Goldberg, 1978) is one common instrument whose criterion validity has been established for several different forms.

Concurrent and predictive validity

There are two main types of criterion validity. The first, concurrent validity, is established when the measure and criterion are measured at the same time. For example, a sample of general practice patients complete the GHQ and are given a structured interview for psychiatric diagnosis (e.g. the Present State Examination (PSE; Wing *et al*, 1974)). The classification of the patients on the PSE is the criterion against which the GHQ is to be validated. In developing an instrument, various cut-off scores will be explored to determine which provides the maximum discrimination between the known groups.

The second aspect of criterion validity is predictive validity, where the criterion is measured later. In psychiatry, measures with predictive validity are typically used to determine a person's likely response to treatment (e.g. the Newcastle Scale for Response to ECT; Kerr *et al*, 1974) or the course of illness (e.g. the Kendrick Battery for Dementia; Kendrick, 1985). Usually one expects the content of the test to be related to the outcome but this is not necessarily so. Nonetheless the content of tests with predictive validity is often determined by the causal models espoused by researchers.

Specificity and sensitivity

Criterion validity is often presented in terms of the specificity and sensitivity of the test. These terms are best explained by referring to Table 8.2, which shows the distribution of cases falling in the cells of a 2 × 2 table produced by allocating them according to whether they exceed the cut-off score of the test and meet the validating criterion.

There are four possible states:

(a) true positive, those defined as positive by both test and criterion
(b) true negative, those defined as negative by both test and criterion
(c) false positive, those incorrectly defined as positive by the test
(d) false negative, those incorrectly defined as negative by the test.

TABLE 8.2
The relationship between scores and their frequencies achieved on a test and classification by an independent criterion

Test	Criterion 1	0
1	True positive *a*	False positive *b*
0	False negative *c*	True negative *d*

$$\text{Sensitivity } (\%) = \frac{a}{a+c} \times 100\%$$

$$\text{Specificity } (\%) = \frac{d}{b+d} \times 100\%$$

$$\text{Base rate } (\%) = \frac{a+c}{a+b+c+d} \times 100\%$$

Scores can be assigned to two categories: 1, when the subject exceeds the cut-off score of the test or the criterion; and 0, when the subject fails to meet the cut-off score or the criterion. The frequencies in four cells are shown as *a*, *b*, *c* and *d*. They can be used to determine the specificity and sensitivity of the test as shown.

The sensitivity of the test is defined as the proportion of positive cases correctly identified. The specificity of the test is the proportion of negative cases identified. These parameters can be modified by altering the cut-off scores. In practice the specificity and sensitivity are determined by the degree to which the scores of cases and non-cases overlap, and the base rate. The base rate is the proportion of true positives in the population. It is important to note that tests developed for application in a given population are not valid for populations with a different base rate. For example, a test developed to predict compliance with drug regimes in psychiatric out-patients will not be valid for a general practice population.

Example: suicide risk in attempted suicides (Pallis et al, 1982, 1984)

Pallis and his colleagues developed scales to predict successful suicide in people who had attempted suicide. In the first study they coded a pool of 203 items that they thought might discriminate between attempted suicide and suicide groups. Data were collected from 151 attempted suicide and 75 suicide patients, a base rate of 34%. After discarding items with poor reliability and infrequent use, 54 items were left for statistical analysis using a discriminant function technique. Pallis and his colleagues derived two scales, of 6 and 18 items. We discuss only the six-item scale.

When this scale was applied to the sample of cases, the best possible cut-off score was capable of correctly classifying 81% of the suicides (61 out of 75) and 84% of the attempted suicides. The purpose of the second study was to test the predictive validity of the scale. Data were collected from 1263 attempted suicides who were followed up for two years. There was a total of 15 suicides in two years, a base rate of 1.18%. The scale correctly classified 60% of these cases. On the other hand, 26% of the attempted suicides were misclassified. This illustrates the influence of the base rate, even in settings where the population characteristics are likely to be very similar. As the authors note, using the scale as a method for detecting suicides for further treatment has severe practical limitations, as one would be overwhelmed by attempted suicides who do not require treatment.

Cross-validation

It is always important to cross-validate a test, that is, to establish whether the test maintains criterion validity when applied to another sample. In most cases the cross-validation takes place in a sample very similar to the original sample, but some published tests have their criterion validity established over a number of populations and the details are published in their manuals.

Checklist for criterion validity

▷ Define the criterion you are interested in very carefully.
▷ Does this match the established criterion of the tests?
▷ Under what conditions was criterion validity established?
   Do they correspond to your conditions?
▷ Over what range of conditions has the criterion validity been established? Is there evidence that it is robust?

Construct validity

Many things which we wish to measure in psychiatry have no single criterion or a content that is entirely determined. In this case the construct validity of the measure must be investigated. Unlike criterion validity, construct validity is not measurable in a single operation or study and evidence for the construct validity must be obtained through a series of inter-related studies. "Construct validity is evaluated by investigating what qualities a test measures, i.e., by demonstrating that certain explanatory constructs account to some degree for the performance on the test" (American Psychological Association, 1954). The construct validity of the test is therefore intimately connected with the theory which underpins the test. For example, Eysenck's well known construct of neuroticism (Eysenck, 1970) contains many predictions about what variables should be associated with each other.

No one variable uniquely validates Eysenck's construct, but the pattern of observed inter-relations obtained over the years provides convincing evidence that such a construct exists and is useful. Intelligence is another well known construct for which there is persuasive evidence.

In order to establish construct validity the theoretical relationships between variables must be specified unambiguously; this will include exploration of potentially confounding variables (alternative explanations). Next the empirical relationships between the variables must be explored and data obtained. Lastly the collected evidence must be weighed and assimilated, and decisions about the validity of the construct must be made.

The central feature of construct validity is the explication of the theoretical construct. Cook & Campbell (1979) give four tests which can be applied to determine whether a construct has validity.

(a) Do independent variables change dependent variables in the direction and manner predicted by the theory?
(b) Do the independent variables fail to alter measures of related but different constructs?
(c) Do the proposed dependent variables tap items that they are meant to measure?
(d) Is it true that the dependent measures are not dominated by irrelevant factors?

Convergent and divergent validity

In classic psychometric technique, construct validity can be determined by establishing convergent and divergent validity. Convergent validity is established when measures that are predicted to be associated (because they measure the same thing) are found to be related. Divergent validity is established when the measures successfully discriminate between other measures of unrelated constructs. For example, one would expect that different measures of abnormal illness behaviour (AIB; Pilowsky, 1969) would be related (correlated) but that they would not be related to measures of neuroticism, a construct which is supposedly independent. If the AIB measures are correlated with neuroticism then one might have doubts as to the validity of the construct of AIB because neuroticism is well established as a construct and it could be argued that it is in some senses more fundamental than AIB. A case example of using neuroticism and AIB, as measured by the Illness Behaviour Questionnaire (IBQ), is given by Zonderman *et al* (1985).

Example: construct validity of the IBQ

Pilowsky (1969) proposed that people who have inappropriate or maladaptive ways of responding to their health could be said to exhibit

AIB. This category was said to include the more traditional concepts such as hysteria, hypochondriasis and conversion reaction. As a consequence of his proposal he developed the IBQ to measure AIB. Zonderman *et al* (1985) attempted to replicate Pilowsky's original research on the IBQ (Pilowsky & Spence, 1975) and to confirm the structure of the subscales of the questionnaire. They also explored the construct validity of the IBQ by correlating it with various personality measures. If the IBQ has good construct validity it should not be strongly correlated with personality measures. Zonderman *et al*, however, found that all the subscales of the IBQ were correlated with three separate measures of neuroticism. In contrast there were few correlations with aspects of personality such as extroversion and 'openness'. This pattern of results suggested that the IBQ overlaps considerably with the construct of neuroticism. Zonderman *et al* noted that this might be interpreted as offering support for the construct validity of the IBQ, because neuroticism is known to be related to complaints about bodily symptoms. Against this positive finding must be set the fact that the subscales of the IBQ do not have any demonstrable discriminant validity, that is, they all seem to measure the same thing. Consequently, Zonderman *et al* argue that previous studies that claim to have demonstrated that the IBQ can separate patients with chronic pain (presumed to be without an organic cause) from other patients are open to reinterpretation. It is possible that the higher scores on the IBQ might represent truthful responses by a person seeking help for bodily complaints which worry him. At present it would seem that the interpretation of IBQ scores is far from clear.

Checklist for construct validity

▷ Is there a theoretical rationale that underpins the measure you are interested in? Is it well articulated so that predictions about the relationships between measures are made?

▷ Is there evidence of a consistent pattern of findings involving different researchers, methods, populations and other theoretical structures over time?

Evaluating negative evidence – alternative explanations

▷ The measure lacks validity as a measure of the construct.

▷ The theoretical framework is incorrect.

▷ The procedure used to test the relationship was faulty.

▷ There is low construct validity because the other variables were measured unreliably.

A note on face validity

'Face validity' denotes the least technical type of validity. A test or measure has face validity if it is judged to measure what it is supposed to measure. There is no way of determining the face validity of a test using statistical methods. It is determined by whether the researcher and his/her colleagues agree that the measure looks as if it is measuring what it is supposed to measure. High face validity can be both an advantage and a disadvantage. It is probable that patients will be more co-operative if they can see that the test is actually measuring something of relevance to them. On the other hand tests with high face validity may make the purpose of the test so obvious that it is easy for the patient to dissimulate.

Reliability

The traditional concept of reliability is concerned with the repeatability of measurement and by implication its vulnerability to error. A common assumption is that a measure is intrinsically reliable or unreliable under all conditions, but it is possible for a test to be highly reliable under one condition and very unreliable under another. Indeed, for certain purposes it is desirable for measures to have this mixed combination of reliabilities. A reliability coefficient is a statement about how far the measure is reproducible in a given set of conditions. The basic procedure for establishing reliability is to obtain two sets of measurements and compare them, usually by the correlation coefficient, the different reliability coefficients reflecting changes in the conditions under which the measures were obtained. There are several reliability coefficients in common use.

Test–retest reliability

Test–retest reliability is established by administering the measure to a group of subjects on two occasions separated by a designated period of time. A perfectly reliable test would have a correlation of 1.0, indicating that the subjects scored exactly the same on both occasions. This never happens as there are several influences that will change the subject's performance on the second occasion. For example, the person's intrinsic state may have changed, or he/she may be fatigued or bored so that careless errors are made. There might also be practice effects so that the more difficult test items can be solved correctly on the second occasion (a special problem in tests of intellectual ability). If the interval is sufficiently long the person will have matured. A major class of error is known as 'reactivity'. This refers to the process whereby the act of measurement induces a change in the object of measurement. For example, measuring people's attitudes to sexual behaviour may prompt them to reconsider their attitudes and change them. A little reflection will produce numerous other confounding sources of change that the test–retest correlation may tap.

A low test–retest reliability may not mean that the measure is 'poor' but that it is susceptible to one of several influences. Clearly the relevance of test–retest reliability will be determined by the construct being measured. For example, if one is concerned with fluctuations in mood during the day it would be inappropriate to select an instrument with high test–retest reliability. This would indicate that it is relatively stable and possibly insensitive to short-term mood changes. One solution would be to select a measure with good 'alternate forms' reliability or high internal consistency, and low test–retest reliability.

Alternate forms reliability

In alternate forms reliability the same subjects are given different, but equivalent, forms of a test on two occasions. The forms of the measure are carefully developed to ensure equivalence as far as possible. This procedure is especially useful if one suspects that there may be a significant learning effect due to the first administration which would seriously bias a second testing on exactly the same measure. Many tests of intellectual ability have alternate forms and there are several personality questionnaires with alternate forms, for example the Eysenck Personality Inventory (Eysenck & Edwards, 1964). As the tests must be administered on two separate occasions the alternate forms reliability coefficient is subject to the same sources of error as test–retest reliability. On the whole this form of reliability is rarely examined in measuring instruments used in psychiatry.

Internal consistency measures of reliability

This type of reliability focuses on the reproducibility of measurement across different items within a test, that is, reproducibility of content. To establish the internal consistency of a measure, the test is administered once to a pool of subjects and the inter-relationship between items on the test is assessed. There are several methods of establishing internal consistency, including the split-half coefficient, the Kuder–Richardson (K–R 20) method and Cronbach's α. All of these reliability coefficients are obtained by intercorrelating subjects' scores on items within a test. If the test is reliable, that is, has internal consistency, then scores on the items should be positively correlated with each other and the internal consistency coefficients will be high. Simple, non-technical guides to these various methods can be found in introductory psychometric texts (Anastasi, 1968; Carmines & Zeller, 1979; Cronbach, 1970).

Internal consistency overcomes the problems of errors introduced by readministering a test. However, the assumption of internal reliability procedures is that items in the test measure more or less the same thing. Insofar as the items tap different constructs one would expect the internal consistency of the test to be reduced. This of course relates to the notions of construct and content validity, which have already been discussed.

Inter-rater reliability

Many measures in psychiatry cannot be repeated in time and the object of measurement is not a construct which can be sampled in different forms, as

TABLE 8.3
The calculation of reliability coefficients for a two-point category scale

	Rater 1		
	1	*0*	
Rater 2			
1	a	b	p_1
0	c	d	q_1
	p_2	q_2	

Raw agreement $= a + d$

Agreement coefficient $= \dfrac{a + d}{a + b + c + d}$

$$\varkappa = \frac{(a + d - p_1 \cdot p_2 - q_1 \cdot q_2)}{(1 - p_1 \cdot p_2 - q_1 \cdot q_2)}$$

Example: two raters might be asked to determine whether a symptom is present (1) or absent (0) in a patient. The letters in the cells are the proportion of frequencies in the cell calculated as a proportion of the total number of observations: $p_1 = a + b$; $q_1 = c + d$; $p_2 = a + c$; $q_2 = b + d$. The calculation of three possible coefficients is shown. The raw agreement and agreement coefficients are easy to calculate, but they do not take into account the probability that the observers will agree by chance. This probability is included in the calculation of $\varkappa$ (kappa).

is required for a measure of internal consistency. The paramount example of this is a diagnostic interview, where a person's mental state will need to be examined at a particular time. Similar problems arise when the overt behaviour of a person has to be sampled as, for example, in the Clifton Assessment Procedures for the Elderly (CAPE; Gilleard & Pattie, 1979). When this problem arises reliability can be assessed by comparing the ratings of two independent observers to determine the extent to which they agree in their observations. There are a number of statistics that are used to compute reliability, and these are shown in Table 8.3.

Agreement on the total score, achieved by summing all the items on a rating scale, is often computed in the form of a correlation coefficient. This will give an estimate of the global reliability of the measure but it is possible to investigate the reliability of the scale in much more detail by calculating the reliability for each item using one of the measures in Table 8.3. This will enable the investigator to determine which aspects of behaviour are poorly defined or difficult to discriminate. This may form a basis for revising the rating scale or improving the training of raters. Generally speaking a reliability measure based on $\varkappa$ is to be recommended because it takes into account the fact that raters can agree by chance. Hall (1974) provides a good worked example of $\varkappa$. (Gamsu (1986) notes that Hall's calculations contain errors and she and Jackson (1983) have developed non-proprietory computer programs for calculating $\varkappa$ which will run on most microcomputers.)

Which reliability coefficient?

Just because studies of the reliability of an instrument have been published, it does not mean that it can be automatically used as a research instrument. Firstly one must assess the type of reliability that has been established and the conditions under which it was examined. This must be compared with the requirements of the planned research. Consider an instrument developed to measure anxiety that is known to have high test–retest reliability, and you wish to measure change in a pool of subjects after they have been given a drug. If there is no change in their score, how should this be interpreted? The two major alternative explanations are that the drug is ineffective or that the instrument is insensitive to change. Knowing that there is a high test–retest correlation would mean that the latter explanation could not be eliminated. In this case it would seem that the scale is designed to measure the enduring trait of anxiety rather than a transient condition or state of anxiety. In practice it would be necessary to select a measure with *low* test–retest reliability but with high internal consistency. In this example we can see the link between reliability and validity. The selection of a test that is sensitive to change will be facilitated if it has already been established that the test is sensitive to various experimental manipulations that are known to alter anxiety, that is, the test's construct validity has been investigated and established.

Secondly it cannot be assumed that because reliability has been ascertained in a previous study, it 'carries over' to other studies. This is particularly true of studies that involve direct observation of behaviour (including interviewer rating scales). In these studies the measuring instrument is the observer, not the scale itself, and it is necessary to ensure that the observers are suitably trained in the definitions of criterion behaviour used by the scale. Even when it has been demonstrated that two observers can reach high levels of agreement during training, it must not be assumed that this reliability will be maintained over the period of study. It is always necessary to conduct reliability probes during the study by sampling the ratings of two or more observers. The picture is further complicated in direct observational studies, as it is possible for the observers to remain highly reliable, as assessed by inter-rater agreement, but yet to drift from the original criteria. Under certain conditions it is possible for observers to be highly reliable but *inaccurate*. This phenomenon of 'observer drift' has been studied by behavioural psychologists and it is known to be influenced by the expectations the observers have about the subjects. Therefore in research involving direct observation, considerable care must be taken to ensure that reliability and accuracy are maintained throughout the study (Hartman, 1982, 1984).

Checklist for reliability

▷ What types of reliability have been established for the measure?
▷ Under what conditions were the reliabilities established? For example, what groups of people were tested, and when and where were they tested?

▷ How closely do your conditions correspond to the original ones?
▷ Do you need to establish reliability for measures in your study? This will almost certainly be necessary for studies involving direct observations of patients.

The concept of generalisability

The astute reader may now be aware that the two concepts of validity and reliability are interwoven. They both relate to the wider question of how far one can make a general statement about the data collected. In other words, given that one has collected data in a certain form, how far is one entitled to generalise from it to other conditions? For example, one would have little confidence in observations collected by a single observer, but consistent data collected by several observers would give confidence that the phenomenon existed in some sense. On the other hand, a measure with predictive validity would enable a general statement about behaviour across time to be made. In both of these examples we are generalising from one set of observations to another and we have some measure of confidence in these generalisations as provided by reliability and validity coefficients.

One advantage of the concept of generalisability is that it forces one to think about the type of generalised statements which one would like to be able to make at the end of a study. The purpose of most research is to provide additional information about a problem that will extend beyond the particular study. Table 8.4 outlines the different domains of generalisability described by Cronbach *et al* (1972) and indicates the sort of questions that one needs to ask about a study.

TABLE 8.4
The main facets of generalisability theory and the typical questions considered

Main facets	Typical questions
Observers/scorers	Can the results be extended across different observers, e.g. interviewers, or test scorers, e.g. independent markers of an IQ test?
Time	Are the data consistent on different occasions of measurement?
Settings	Are the observations in one setting consistent with observations from another setting? How far can one generalise between the various settings?
Subjects	How far can the observations be generalised from one person to another?
Item/behaviour	How do the items on a test, or different behaviours, relate to each other?

The facets correspond to traditional notions of reliability and validity. For example the time facet corresponds to test–retest reliability. Cronbach, who introduced generalisability theory, demonstrated how it was possible to consider more than one facet at a time by using the statistical methods of analysis of variance.

Conclusions

The selection of an appropriate set of measures for research requires very careful consideration. Just because a test or rating scale has been published does not ensure that it is psychometrically appropriate for all uses. Readers are cautioned to be aware of the face validity of measures – the notion that if a measure looks good it is good. The selection of an appropriate measure requires very careful specification of the research hypothesis and possible alternative rival hypotheses. This is usually achieved only after reflection and discussion with experienced colleagues. Once the central issues have been decided it becomes clearer what measurement is required. At this stage a literature search may reveal that certain instruments have been repeatedly used. Some of these studies should be carefully investigated to document the known details of reliability and validity of the instrument. It is also useful to contact others who have used the instruments to obtain their opinion and expertise. Finally when a measure is selected, plans must be drawn up to determine what aspects of reliability or validity will need to be monitored in the planned study. On occasions the researchers will be left with no option other than to develop their own measure or to modify a previously published instrument. In that case extensive provision for the study of the reliability and validity of the instrument must be made.

References

AMERICAN PSYCHOLOGICAL ASSOCIATION (1954) Technical recommendations for psychological tests and diagnostic techniques. *Psychological Bulletin*, (suppl. 51, part 2), 1–38.

ANASTASI, A. (1968) *Psychological Testing* (3rd edn). London: MacMillan.

BECK, A. T., WARD, C. H., MENDELSON, M., *et al* (1961) An inventory for measuring depression. *Archives of General Psychiatry*, **4**, 561–571.

CARMINES, E. G. & ZELLER, R. A. (1979) *Reliability and Validity Assessment*. Beverly Hills: Sage Publications.

COOK, T. D. & CAMPBELL, D. T. (1979) *Quasi-experimentation. Design and Analysis Issues for Field Settings*. Chicago: Rand McNally.

CRONBACH, L. (1970) *Essentials of Psychological Testing* (3rd edn). New York: Harper and Row.

——, GLESER, G. C., NANDA, H., *et al* (1972) *The Dependability of Behavioral Measures*. New York: Wiley.

EYSENCK, H. J. (1970) *Structure of Human Personality* (3rd edn). London: Hodder.

—— & EDWARDS, S. (1964) *The Eysenck Personality Questionnaire*. Windsor: NFER/Nelson.

GAMSU, C. V. (1986) Calculating reliability measures for ordinal data. *British Journal of Clinical Psychology*, **25**, 307–308.

GILLEARD, C. & PATTIE, A. (1979) *Clifton Assessment Procedures for the Elderly*. Windsor: NFER/Nelson.

GOLDBERG, D. (1978) *Manual of the General Health Questionnaire*. Slough: National Foundation for Educational Research.

HALL, J. N. (1974) Inter-rater reliability of ward rating scales. *British Journal of Psychiatry*, **125**, 248–255.

HARTMAN, D. P. (1982) *Using Observers to Study Behavior*. New directions for methodology in social and behavioral science, no. 14. San Francisco: Jossey-Bass.

—— (1984) Assessment strategies. In *Single Case Experimental Designs. Strategies for Studying Behavior Change* (2nd edn) (eds D. H. Barlow & M. Hersen). New York: Pergamon.

JACKSON, P. R. (1983) An easy to use BASIC program for agreement amongst many raters. *British Journal of Clinical Psychology*, **22**, 145–146.

KENDRICK, D. C. (1985) *Kendrick Cognitive Tests for the Elderly*. Windsor: NFER/Nelson.

KERR, T. A., ROTH, M. & SCHAPIRA, K. (1974) Prediction of outcome in anxiety states and depressive illness. *British Journal of Psychiatry*, **124**, 125–133.

PALLIS, D. J., BARRACLOUGH, B. M., LEVEY, A. B., *et al* (1982) Estimating suicide risk among attempted suicides: I. The development of new clinical scales. *British Journal of Psychiatry*, **141**, 37–44.

——, GIBBONS, J. S. & PIERCE, D. W. (1984) Estimating suicide risk among attempted suicides: II. Efficiency of predictive scales after the attempt. *British Journal of Psychiatry*, **144**, 139–148.

PILOWSKY, I. (1969) Abnormal illness behaviour. *British Journal of Medical Psychology*, **42**, 347–351.

—— & SPENCE, N. D. (1975) Patterns of illness behaviour in patients with intractable pain. *Journal of Psychosomatic Research*, **19**, 279–287.

WILLIAMS, P., TARNOPOLSKY, A. & HAND, D. (1980) Case definition and identification in psychiatric epidemiology: review and assessment. *Psychological Medicine*, **10**, 101–114.

WING, J. K., COOPER, J. E. & SARTORIUS, N. (1974) *The Measurement and Classification of Psychiatric Symptoms*. London: Cambridge University Press.

ZIGMOND, A. S. & SNAITH, R. P. (1983) The Hospital Anxiety and Depression Scale. *Acta Psychiatrica Scandinavica*, **67**, 361–370.

ZONDERMAN, A. B., HEFT, M. W. & COSTA, P. T. (1985) Does the illness behavior questionnaire measure abnormal illness behavior? *Health Psychology*, **4**, 425–436.

Further reading

CARMINES, E. G. & ZELLER, R. A. (1979) *Reliability and Validity Assessment*. Beverly Hills: Sage Publications. This small text provides an excellent introduction to traditional psychometric concepts, is invaluable, and contains good examples of how the various formulae are applied.

LEMKE, E. & WIERSMA, W. (1976) *Principles of Psychological Assessment*. Chicago: Rand McNally. This is more extensive than Carmines & Zeller's text, but it is beautifully laid out with excellent examples. Each chapter has test questions appended to it. Recommended to readers who wish to grapple with the more technical aspects of psychometrics.

WIGGINS, J. S. (1973) *Personality and Prediction: Principles of Personality Assessment*. Reading, Massachusetts: Addison-Wesley. This text is a comprehensive coverage of the literature and concepts up to 1973. Wiggins provides an excellent review of the field. In particular there is an elegant introduction to generalisability theory.

NUNALLY, J. C. (1978) *Psychometric Theory* (2nd edn). New York: McGraw-Hill. This is one of the standard texts on psychometrics. It is comprehensive and contains advanced coverage of psychometric theory and practice.

BENNETT, A. E. & RICHIE, K. (1975) *Questionnaires in Medicine. A Guide to their Design and Use*. Oxford: Oxford University Press. Exactly what it says it is: an easy-to-read guide to the design and use of questionnaires. It also contains reviews of the most popular questionnaires, but is now a little out of date.

9 Rating instruments in psychiatric research

BRIAN FERGUSON and PETER TYRER

Rating scales are the most common measuring instruments in clinical psychiatric research and there are few projects that are carried out in the field of clinical psychiatry that do not use them. They have many different applications, but screening, diagnosis, and the measurement of severity and change are among the most important. For a rating scale to be useful it needs to be both valid and reliable (see Chapter 8) and the aspiring research worker needs to be familiar with these terms and their measurement before choosing a rating scale for a project. Unfortunately, although reliability can be recorded satisfactorily in most psychiatric research, there are few instances when a scale can be regarded as having proven validity. However, for research purposes a sufficient approximation to validity can be made to be useful, and the research worker needs to decide what type of validity is required for the purposes of the project. The literature on rating instruments in psychiatry is a rather confusing one and it is sometimes extremely difficult to find the right measure for a particular purpose. This chapter and Chapters 10 and 11 attempt to find a way through the rating-scale maze. This inevitably involves some short cuts and some areas of endeavour are not covered fully. However, for these areas the reader is referred to more detailed texts.

Choosing a rating instrument

A flow chart (Fig. 9.1) can be used to indicate the stages involved in choosing an instrument for rating in psychiatric research. Some of the questions may appear self-evident, but they need to be asked if expensive mistakes are to be avoided.

Nature of measurement

Although rating scales are often essential in psychiatric research they are not always necessary. It is sometimes possible to obtain the information

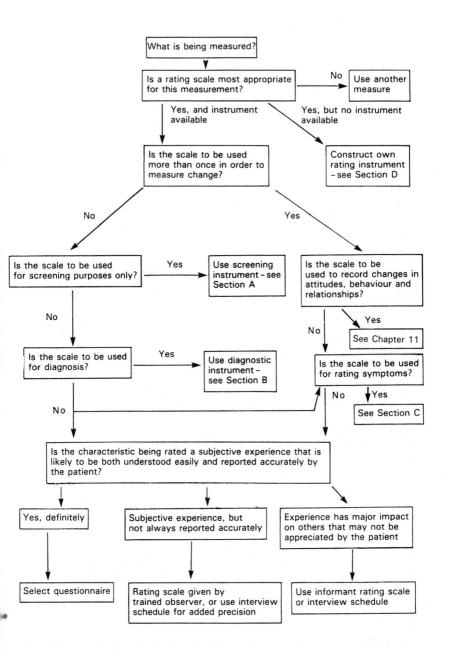

Fig. 9.1   Flow chart for selection of rating instruments in psychiatric research

contained in a rating scale more easily by other means. For example, the research worker might be interested in the incidence of relapse in manic–depressive psychosis following different treatments. Although this information can be obtained by prospective use of rating scales, the simple recording of data such as admissions to hospital and numbers of attempted and successful suicides may be of equal or greater value. In research terms, all data derived from rating scales are regarded as 'soft' whereas statistics such as those recording mortality are 'hard'. A study which showed that the suicide rate following one type of treatment was significantly lower than that following another would, therefore, carry greater weight than one that merely indicated a quantitative change in symptoms recorded by a rating scale.

In most instances, however, there is no other independent measure that could replace the rating scale in psychiatric research. Most psychiatric information is predominantly descriptive and the main purpose of the rating scale is to convert this into quantifiable numerical data that are susceptible to statistical analysis. Sometimes in this technological age all numerical data are regarded as superior to descriptions, but a historical perspective of psychiatry shows this view to be incorrect. The research worker need not feel ashamed about recording findings in descriptive terms only. Most advances in psychiatry have come through the dissemination of written and verbal material, and its conversion into numerical data would have had little impact. In general, when breaking entirely new ground it is probably wise to avoid using rating scales, at least in pilot studies, because of the dangers that they may restrict inquiry and fail to detect important changes.

Measurement of change

It is important for the research worker to ask at an early stage whether a rating instrument is to be used to measure change. Although many rating instruments can be used repeatedly to record changes, many are cumbersome and relatively insensitive. In recent years more attention has been paid to the sensitivity of scales in detecting small changes and, provided that sensitivity is not gained at the expense of specificity, this is an obvious advantage. The other major issue is one of practicality. An excellent instrument that takes four hours to administer is not going to be appropriate to give to a patient at weekly intervals. When reading the original papers on rating scales it is useful to find out how long the instrument takes to administer by a trained assessor. Unfortunately, this information is sometimes missing but it is essential when planning a study.

If the instrument is to be used only once, as for example in many diagnostic and epidemiological studies, or for screening purposes, the length is not so important, but even so, may become a critical factor. In an epidemiological study the subjects interviewed will often have little or no disorder and will be unhappy about answering a long series of questions to which the answers are predominantly negative. This problem can be overcome by paying subjects to be interviewed, as is common in many epidemiological studies in the United States, but this introduces another factor that could produce bias.

Rating scales for screening purposes, diagnosis, and recording changes in symptoms are the most common in psychiatry and each of these is given a separate section in this chapter (see Fig. 9.1). Because much of psychiatry is concerned with more subtle changes, particularly those of attitudes in relationships, a separate group of instruments has been developed that examines these characteristics. These are discussed in Chapter 10, and have their own special advantages as well as problems.

Source of information

At an early stage it is important to ask whether the measurement being requested is more likely to be better reported by the subject or patient or by an independent observer. With increasing psychometric sophistication and development of long interview schedules, the view is gaining ground that questionnaires are the poor relations in the rating-scale family, and that carefully constructed structured interviews will provide more valid and reliable data. This is untrue, because the most important issue is the nature of the information. Thus, if the research worker wanted to find out patients' attitudes towards admission to, for example, a psychiatric unit in a general hospital compared with a traditional mental hospital, it would be preferable to do this through the construction of an unbiased questionnaire rather than a structured interview schedule or any form of observer rating scale. At the other end of the spectrum, a questionnaire for depressive symptoms would be totally inappropriate for a population of patients with depressive stupor.

If the characteristic is a subjective experience that is clear cut and can be reported accurately, then a questionnaire is preferable; if it is likely to be distorted or have other difficulties in its expression then an observer rating scale may be appropriate. Most psychiatric disorders have both a subjective and 'objective' component, including behavioural disturbance and changes in relationships that may be more noticeable to other people. In such circumstances it is perfectly appropriate to give both a self-rating scale and an observer-rated instrument. In practice, the results of these often correlate highly and it is unwise to include too many scales that are attempting to measure the same changes. If the characteristic being rated is one that has a major impact on other people and may not always be fully appreciated by the patient (e.g. personality disorder) it may be more appropriate to rely on independent information from a close informant rather than the subject.

Structured interview schedules with either subject or informant usually give improved reliability, but should not be assumed to carry increased validity. They have become particularly popular in the United States since the introduction of DSM–III (American Psychiatric Association, 1980). Most of these instruments focus on the operational criteria in DSM–III (and

DSM–III–R; American Psychiatric Association, 1987) and this can be particularly helpful when the operational criteria are good ones and based on good experimental data. However, many of the DSM–III operational criteria can be described as only intelligent guesswork and for these the perceived advantages of interview schedules are suspect.

If the research worker follows the flow chart shown in Fig. 9.1, it is likely that a suitable instrument is already available for the subject required by the investigator. If, after exhaustive inquiry, no instrument is found to exist, then it is reasonable to construct one specifically for the study in question. This procedure has many pitfalls and requires much hard work. It is discussed in Section D.

In both this chapter and Chapter 10 some of the more frequently used rating scales and other measuring instruments are listed and their strengths and weaknesses indicated. The list of references at the end of the chapter will direct the interested reader to a published description of the instrument in addition to providing further information on subsequent reliability and validity studies. The text discusses some of the major scales in more detail but presupposes that the reader already has a specific research project under consideration and knows what is to be measured. It is important to bear in mind that although most instruments have been devised for a specific purpose, their use need not always be restricted in this way.

Section A. Screening: the detection of general emotional and psychiatric morbidity

Detecting psychiatric morbidity in community samples has been a source of considerable interest over many years (Table 9.1). The earliest attempts (Clouston, 1911) were based on interviews by psychiatrists, which are obviously costly and time consuming. More latterly, self-administered screening questionnaires have been developed so that large numbers of people can be interviewed economically. One of the most widely known is the General Health Questionnaire (GHQ) developed by Goldberg (1972) at the Maudsley Hospital, which detects non-psychotic psychiatric ill health. The 60-item version takes 10–15 minutes to complete and has satisfactory sensitivity and specificity. A high score indicates the likely presence of psychiatric morbidity but does not provide a diagnosis. The instrument tends to miss patients suffering from psychotic disorders and those who are inclined to behave defensively when filling in questionnaires. Long-standing neurotic patients who are in a period of partial remission of symptoms may also be missed because the questionnaire asks them to compare their recent state of mind with their ''usual'' state. The GHQ has been used in a variety of settings including community studies, social and occupational research, and psychiatric morbidity associated with physical disorders (Shepherd *et al*, 1981).

TABLE 9.1
General morbidity scales

Name	Authors	No. of items	Main features
General Health Questionnaire (GHQ)	Goldberg (1972)	60 (12) (20) (30)	Self-administered screening tool Questions refer to past 4 weeks Detects non-psychotic psychiatric illness Cut-off point of 11 (60 item) and 5 (30 item) identifies a case 4-point scale
Hopkins Symptom Checklist (HSC)	Parloff *et al* (1954), elaborated by Frank (1957)	58 (90) (72) (64) (35)	Self-administered Refers to symptoms during previous week 4-point scale Used to measure psychiatric improvement in neurotic population
Health Opinion Survey (HOS) (MacMillan Index)	MacMillan (1957), Leighton *et al* (1963), abbreviated version by Spiro *et al* (1972)	75 13	Self-administered Questions deal with psychophysiological complaints and social relationships Discriminates between known patients and general population For use in epidemiological studies 3-point scales
Symptom Sign Inventory (SSI)	Foulds (1965)	80	Administered by trained interviewer Yes/no answers Principal use is as diagnostic instrument but can be used for case identification in epidemiological studies
Personal Disturbance Scale	Foulds & Hope (1968)	20	
Iowa Structured Psychiatric Interview	Tsuang *et al* (1980)	235	Extensive personal and family history section Administered by trained non-medical interviewer Designed for epidemiological research in general population 20 core screening questions for mania, schizophrenia, depression and neurosis

The Health Opinion Survey (HOS) was a screening test developed to detect psychoneurotic and related disorders in the Sterling County Studies (MacMillan, 1957). The original form consisted of 75 questions, the central core of 15 being derived from the army's neuropsychiatric adjunct, which had been used to help identify psychiatric illness in new recruits. The scale is heavily biased towards somatic symptoms and some doubt has been cast on its validity in view of the low correlation between HOS scores and clinical assessment of severity (Leighton *et al*, 1963). An abbreviated version called the MacMillan Index however has been developed by Spiro *et al* (1972), who consider that it clearly discriminates between psychiatric patients and the rest of the population from which they come. They suggest that it is a good screening instrument for epidemiological studies but is not of value as a diagnostic tool.

The Iowa Structured Psychiatric Interview (Tsuang *et al*, 1980) was also designed for epidemiological research in the general population. It assesses current psychiatric symptoms utilising 20 core screening questions for major psychiatric syndromes: depression, mania, schizophrenia, and neurosis. It also elicits details of social, alcohol and drug history, previous physical, psychiatric and family history, and a rating of present behaviour. It is administered by trained non-medical personnel and is not suitable for interviews of patients for clinical purposes, but it is structured so that information on present symptoms is sought before knowledge of past history is obtained, thus providing for an important element of 'blind' assessment. It was originally developed for the large epidemiological Iowa 500 project (Tsuang & Winokur, 1975) and has been shown to have good validity and inter-rater reliability in respect of the mania, depression and schizophrenia items, but less so for the neurosis items. The behaviour ratings were considered to be too unreliable for research work. It has been especially recommended for use in long-term follow-up and family studies of affective disorders and schizophrenia.

The Hopkins Symptom Checklist (Parloff *et al*, 1954) differs from the previously described instruments insofar as it was originally developed to measure clinical improvement during the course of psychotherapy. The total score on the 64-item version provides an overall assessment of emotional distress in terms of five dimensions: somatisation, obsessive–compulsive, interpersonal sensitivity, depression, and anxiety. Factor analysis of the 90-item version increases the yield to eight clinically meaningful dimensions, including retarded depression, agitated depression, anger, hostility, phobic anxiety and psychoticism. The scores of items comprising individual factors can be summed and then divided by the number of items rated by each dimension. Mean scores range from one to four and it has been suggested that a score greater than 1.75 in any of these measures may indicate the need for psychiatric attention. The checklist has been used both as a screening procedure for emotional distress and as an assessment of change in various clinical populations including obstetric and gynaecological patients (Rickels *et al*, 1976), family planning clinics, psychotherapeutic settings and psycho-pharmacology research work (Lipman *et al*, 1965).

Section B. Psychiatric classification and diagnosis

In order to use these schedules (Table 9.2) wisely, it is important to appreciate the differences between allocating cases to descriptive classes and the application of a clinical diagnosis. Diagnosis distinguishes one disease from another and has implications for treatment, course and aetiology. Assignation of a case to a particular class on the basis of the presence of one or more symptoms or signs that define that class has no such implications *per se*. Many interview schedules tend to focus on either classification or diagnosis as a primary

TABLE 9.2
Diagnostic schedules

Name	Authors	Main features
Schedule for Affective Disorders and Schizophrenia (SADS)	Endicott & Spitzer (1978)	Interview designed to elicit information necessary for making RDC diagnosis Diagnosis is either present or absent Takes 1½–2 hours to complete Three versions: SADS, SADS-L and SADS-C Requires trained psychiatrist, psychologist or social worker
National Institute of Mental Health Diagnostic Interview Schedule (NIMH DIS)	Robins *et al* (1979)	Designed to be used with Feighner's criteria –may be scored according to RDC Structured fixed phrasing interview, lasting 1–1½ hours No diagnostic heirarchy imposed Diagnosis present, probable or absent Trained clinicians or non-clinicians
Brief Psychiatric Rating Scale (BPRS)	Overall & Gorham (1962)	Semistructured interview, lasting 20–30 minutes Yields 8 phenomenological classes Can be used for evaluating nature and extent of therapeutic effect More appropriate for research on in-patients
Present State Examination and CATEGO Program (PSE)	Wing *et al* (1974)	Structured mental state interview which does not use historical information Provides descriptive symptom and syndrome profiles. Requires trained clinician CATEGO computer program classifies mental state data (can be compared to ICD groups)
In-patient Multidimensional Psychiatric Scale (IMPS)	Lorr *et al* (1963)	Covers neurotic and psychotic symptomatology Semistructured 1-hour interview Emphasis on present state Yields 12 syndromes (defined as a cluster or collection of symptoms and behaviour)
Arbeitsgemeinschaft fur Methodik und Dokumentation der Psychiatrie (AMP)	Angst *et al* (1967)	Instrument for documentation of clinical data including general history, psychiatric case record, and psychopathological and somatic state Based on classical English and German psychopathology Used in German- and French-speaking countries (Serbo-Croatian version also available)
Structured Clinical Interview for DSM–III (SCID)	Spitzer *et al* (1985)	Designed to yield specific DSM–III diagnosis Axes I and II Trained clinical personnel Three versions depending on the clinical population to be interviewed

objective, but in view of the close relationship between the two, it is often possible to apply a dual purpose when additional information is available.

The Present State Examination (PSE; Wing *et al*, 1974) is a structured interview designed to identify certain symptomatic and behavioural phenomena and to provide precise rules for classification, so that an individual with a given pattern of symptoms will always be allocated to the same clinical grouping. It was developed to enhance the reliability of psychiatric diagnosis and therefore to be used as a research tool. The principal value of the PSE has been to standardise the description of the mental state of patients from differing cultures and backgrounds in order to allow clear comparisons of research findings (Cooper *et al*, 1972; World Health Organization, 1973). Because it yields scores in various areas of psychopathology it can be used as a measure of change and has been widely applied in the evaluation of treatment programmes. The interview usually records symptoms present during the previous month but the accompanying syndrome checklist can be used to describe symptoms that have been present on previous occasions. Other symptoms are rated on the basis of behaviour, affect and speech during the examination itself and may not therefore reflect the level of symptoms over a prolonged period. The information from the 140 items is used to provide: (a) a symptom score (present or absent/moderate or severe), (b) a syndrome score (symptoms serve to define scores on one of the 20 psychotic syndromes or 16 neurotic syndromes), (c) quantitative subscores derived from syndrome scores, and (d) quantitative total scores, i.e. the sum of the four quantitative subscores. In addition a computer program assigns one out of the 12 CATEGO classes (related to clinical diagnosis). A screening version of the PSE has been developed for use in epidemiological studies. In general the instrument has been found to have very acceptable reliability except in the area of observed behaviour (Wing *et al*, 1974). A further discussion of reliability and validity in patients with a functional psychiatric disorder can be found in an article by Luria & Berry (1979). Van de Hout & Griez (1984) have suggested that the neurotic syndrome scores cannot be used to provide a meaningful subdivision of a clinical neurotic population, especially in the case of obsessive–compulsive neurosis. Reliability is partly achieved through standardised training of raters which should be carried out by established practitioners before the PSE is used. An updated version (SCAN) of the PSE suitable for the forthcoming ICD–10 classification is currently undergoing field trials.

The Schedule for Affective Disorders and Schizophrenia (SADS) is designed to yield diagnosis according to the New York Research Diagnostic Criteria (Endicott & Spitzer, 1978). It uses a hierarchical system to make a diagnosis so that the investigator can omit lower-order diagnostic questions if criteria for a higher-order diagnosis have been met. There are three versions. The regular version (SADS) has two parts, the first of which looks at the current episode and functioning in the week before interview. The second looks at past psychiatric disturbance. The lifetime version (SADS–L) looks at the past and current disturbances, and the SADS–C is the version for measuring change.

The National Institute of Mental Health (NIMH) Diagnostic Interview Schedule (DIS) has been developed for large-scale epidemiological work. Non-clinicians have been found to be as effective as clinicians in rating its items (Hesselbrook *et al*, 1982). The schedule examines both past and current episodes, determines age at onset of diagnosable conditions, number of episodes, length of longest episode and age at last episode. Because it does not impose a hierarchy, more information is obtained than with the SADS. Both instruments can be used to rate DSM–III Axis I (clinical psychiatric syndrome), Axis II (personality disorders) and Axis V (highest level of adaptive functioning, past year). The NIMH DIS can also be used to rate Axis III (physical disorders) but additional information is required by both for Axis IV (severity of psychosocial stressors).

The choice of instrument to be used frequently depends on the level of clinical expertise possessed by the raters. However, there is another factor that needs to be taken into account. The various research diagnostic criteria, although standardised, differ among themselves in respect of the number of criteria required for specific diagnoses. In a study of 166 patients with a clinical diagnosis of schizophrenia, Overall & Hollister (1979) found that while only 26% satisfied the Feighner criteria (Feighner *et al*, 1972) there was disagreement between Research Diagnostic Criteria (Spitzer *et al*, 1975) and Feighner criteria 50% of the time. The investigator therefore needs to know which criteria are suitable for a particular study and should become familiar with them before selecting the appropriate schedule (see Overall & Hollister (1979) for a fuller discussion of this issue).

The reliability and validity of the DIS have been examined in the Epidemiological Catchment Area (ECA) project. Anthony *et al* (1985) found that prevalence rates based on the DIS one-month diagnoses were significantly different from those based on standardised DSM–III diagnoses by psychiatrists. Major depression seems to be diagnosed by lay interviewers less frequently whereas obsessional illness is diagnosed more often. It was noted that although lay interviewers and physicians may agree on the presence of a disorder there is less agreement on the diagnosis (Helzer *et al*, 1985).

An alternative method of investigation is to make DSM–III–R diagnoses directly using the Structured Clinical Interview Schedule (SCID) developed by Spitzer *et al* (1985). The schedule is for use by clinically trained personnel and comes in three versions. The SCID–P is designed for use with in-patients, the SCID–OP for use with out-patients or where a more detailed assessment of psychotic symptoms is not required, and the SCID–NP is designed for use in non-psychiatric patient populations. Each major diagnosis is dealt with by a separate module, so that modules can be used selectively if required in pre-defined populations. Modifications dealing with the severity of specific illnesses (e.g. depression) are available and the schedules allow for the determination of DSM–III Axis I and Axis II diagnoses (SCID–II). They have been prepared in such a way as to satisfy the operational diagnostic criteria according to DSM–III–R. The questions are designed to simulate the clinical diagnostic process and are preceded by an overview of the present illness before going on to consider some past and most present symptoms. Unfortunately, no reliability data on SCID in its several versions are available.

Section C. Instruments primarily used for measuring change in psychopathology

Although most instruments will record a significant change in mental status, some have been developed primarily with this purpose in mind. The Brief Psychiatric Rating Scale (BPRS; Overall, 1974) was originally developed as a rapidly administered, semistructured interview to evaluate treatment response in drug studies. It covers most in-patient psychopathology and uses information obtained and behaviour observed during the interview. Cluster-analysis techniques have identified eight phenomenological types: florid thinking disorder, withdrawn disorganised thinking disturbances, paranoid hostile/suspiciousness, anxious depression, hostile depression, retarded depression, agitation/excitement, and agitated depression. There is obviously some overlap between these classes and the more commonly used clinical diagnoses but they are not necessarily interchangeable.

The Comprehensive Psychopathological Rating Scale (CPRS) was developed by Åsberg et al (1978) as an instrument for measuring change in levels of psychopathology. Its 65 items cover a wide range of pathology in both psychotic and neurotic conditions largely using non-technical language, and it can easily be administered by trained personnel. Four subscales have been identified for specific areas of pathology: the Brief Anxiety Scale (Tyrer et al, 1984), and the depression (MADRS; Montgomery & Åsberg, 1979), obsessional and schizophrenia scales (Montgomery & Montgomery, 1980). The inter-rater reliability of the CPRS has been compared with that of the other continental system, the AMP (Angst et al, 1967) (see Table 9.2) and was found to be slightly superior in respect of symptoms but of equal reliability in respect of derived syndrome scales (Maurer et al, 1984).

The Nurses Observation Scale for Inpatient Evaluation (NOSIE–30) is a ward behaviour rating scale that was developed to measure therapeutic change in schizophrenic patients (Honigfeld et al, 1966). Reports on the level of inter-rater reliability have varied (Honigfeld et al, 1966; McMordie & Swint, 1979) on average intraclass correlation between 0.57 and 0.74. Satisfactory reliability is best for the subscales that examine the more easily observed positive items, although male raters tend to be more tolerant and score lower for negative behaviour. It has been shown to have a particular value in selecting and assessing patients for treatment programmmes and has been used in the development of scales for the assessment of negative and positive symptoms of schizophrenia (Lewine et al, 1983). Thirty items cover three positive factors (personal neatness, social competence and social interest) and three negative factors (manifest psychosis, retardation and irritability) which can be summed for total scores.

TABLE 9.3
Instruments for assessing deficit syndromes and negative symptoms in schizophrenia

Title	Authors	Main features
Quality of Life Scale	Heinrichs et al (1984)	Semistructured interview for deficit syndrome 21 items covering symptoms and functioning during previous 4 weeks Trained clinician, takes 45 minutes Each item scored on 7-point scale Excludes relationships with mental health worker
Rating Scale for Emotional Blunting	Abrams & Taylor (1978)	Clinical interview by psychiatrist 16 items rated Covers affect, behaviour and thought content
Scale for Affective Flattening	Andreasen (1979)	Evaluation of observable phenomena by clinician 4-point rating scale and global scale 9 items rated
Negative Symptom Rating Scale	Iager et al (1985)	10 items 7-point scale Assesses thought processes, volition cognition and affect 15-minute semistructured interview
Scale for Assessment of Negative Symptoms	Andreasen (1982)	30 negative items Total score indicates level of severity 5 subscales of affective blunting, alogia, avolition, apathy, anhedonia, asociality and attentional impairment Not pathognomonic of schizophrenia

Instruments for assessing negative symptoms and deficit states in schizophrenia

Many of the foregoing instruments include items covering negative symptoms, but in general this aspect of psychopathology assessment has been neglected, for operational reasons. For example, the Feighner criteria for schizophrenia exclude emotional blunting because of an inability to achieve satisfactory inter-rater agreement when it is present in a relatively mild form (Feighner et al, 1972). More recently scales have emerged that have achieved better levels of inter-rater reliability (Table 9.3). The rating scale for emotional blunting has an ability to distinguish between schizophrenia and affective disorder but this claim was principally based on a comparison of patients suffering from schizophrenia and hypomania. Andreasen (1979, 1982) has shown that such scales are not likely to be able to differentiate between schizophrenia and the depressive pole of affective disorder. Negative symptoms and deficit states are not synonymous. Blunted affect, for example, may be a pronounced feature during florid psychotic episodes. The Quality of Life Scale (Heinrichs et al, 1984) uses an observational clinical approach to assess symptoms and functioning over a few weeks and attempts to take into account the patient's opportunity for interaction with others.

A standardised rating scale for assessing chronic psychotic patients has been developed by Krawiecka *et al* (1977) and is quick and simple to use. Its principal function so far has been to assess patients for rehabilitation and for evaluating change in drug trials. A unique ten-item Treatment Response Scale (TRS) has been used to assess response to neuroleptic therapy on the basis of retrospective analysis of in-patient hospital records (Csernansky *et al*, 1983).

Rating scales for mania

Beigel *et al* (1971) developed the first scale for use exclusively in manic conditions to provide the clear advantage of reliable use by nursing staff. The items are scored according to intensity and frequency and several forms modified for interview are available (Bech *et al*, 1975; Blackburn, 1977) (see Table 9.4). Two subgroups, elated grandiose and paranoid destructive, can be identified using the ratings and there are 11 co-items which best characterise the severe disturbances. The Rating Scale for Mania (Young *et al*, 1978) and the Bech–Rafaelsen Rating Scale for Mania (Bech *et al*, 1979) appeared roughly at the same time and have little to choose between them. Some items of the Young scale (irritability, speech rate and amount, speech content, and disruptive aggressive behaviour) are weighted in order to compensate for poor co-operation from severely ill patients. The Petterson scale, consisting of seven items, is also a clinician-administered interview (Petterson *et al*, 1973) suitable for longitudinal ratings. Because insight is usually poor, self-rating scales are generally inappropriate in mania, patients' perceptions of their emotional state having very little correlation with those

TABLE 9.4
Rating scales for mania

Name	Authors	Main features
Bech–Rafaelsen Rating Scale for Mania (combined rating scale for mania and depression)	Bech *et al* (1979) Rafaelsen *et al* (1980)	11 items Requires experienced clinical rater Scores based on clinical interview 5-point scale Total score may be used as index of severity, range 0–44
Rating Scale for Mania	Young *et al* (1978)	11 items (4 items receive double weighting) For use by trained rater Total score indicates level of severity
Manic State Rating Scale	Beigel *et al* (1971), modified by Blackburn *et al* (1977)	26 observable items Can be rated by nursing staff 6 of the items useful for measuring change Blackburn version modified for interview use with 2 additional scales

of supervising staff (Platman *et al*, 1969). Nonetheless one such rating scale does exist and is able to differentiate manic patients from depressed patients and normal individuals (Plutchik, 1967).

Depression rating scales

Judging by the extensive literature, the development of rating scales for depression, particularly of the self-report type, has occupied the minds of numerous investigators over many years (Table 9.5). Indeed, Snaith (1981) has called for a moratorium on the production of further depression scales until the existing ones have been fully compared and reassessed. It is a tribute to Max Hamilton that his rating scale has outlived many others and is now recognised as the standard observer rating scale for depression, especially in the assessment of treatment response. Numerous modifications have been made by different authors (Miller *et al*, 1985; Paykel, 1985) and others have used the scale as a basis for the derivation of their own instruments (Bech, 1984). Carroll *et al* (1981) have described a self-rating version which has been shown to be a convenient and reliable alternative (Nasr *et al*, 1984).

The Hamilton Rating Scale for Depression (HRSD; Hamilton, 1960) is not designed as a diagnostic instrument although some studies appear to regard it as one, often using a cut-off score to indicate the presence of a depressive illness. The assessment should be made by a physician using information obtained from all available sources, including a clinical interview of at least half an hour. It was originally suggested that the scale should be rated by two observers and their scores summed to give the final score. In practice this is very difficult to arrange in most research studies, so the single score is simply doubled.

The original scale contained 21 items but this was reduced to 17 because three of them, depersonalisation/derealisation, paranoid and obsessional symptoms, were found to be less common. The fourth item, diurnal variation, was considered to record the form of the illness and not the severity. Most of the items are graded 0–4 although some items, insomnia, gastrointestinal somatic symptoms, genital symptoms, insight, weight loss and general somatic symptoms, are rated 0–2 because it was found difficult to make fine distinctions between them in practice. The limitation on scoring grades was deliberately introduced to prevent a central tendency of scoring. Using Rasch statistics Bech (1984) has suggested that a subset of six HRSD items constitute a one-dimensional measure of change in depressive states and has incorporated them into the Melancholia Scale (MES), which can be used to screen for depression and can categorise illness according to severity.

Much effort has been expended in assessing the shortcomings of the HRSD. Maier & Philipp (1985) have listed the main criticisms as follows: heterogeneous and unstable factor analytic structure, missing general factor, missing course validation and neglect of self-reported feelings of distress in

TABLE 9.5
Depression rating scales

Name	Authors	Mode of administration	No. of items	Main features
Hamilton Rating Scale for Depression (HRSD)	Hamilton (1960)	Clinical interview	21 (17)	Quantifies level of depression but not diagnostic tool
General Practitioner Research Group Depression Scale	Gringras (1980)	Physician rating	11	Used to measure depression in general practice studies
Beck Depression Inventory (BDI)	Beck *et al* (1961)	Self-rating, administered by interview	21 (13)	Measures depth of depression and therefore used as measure of treatment outcome
Middlesex Hospital Questionnaire (MHQ)	Crown & Crisp (1966)	Self-rating	48	6 susbscales used to measure psychoneurotic status: phobic anxiety, obsessional, somatic, hysterical and anxiety
Centre for Epidemiological Studies (CES–D)	Radloff (1977)	Self-report	20	First-stage screening test for depression in epidemiological studies
Hospital Anxiety and Depression Scale (HADS)	Zigmond & Snaith (1983)	Self-rating	14	Detection of anxiety and depression in medical and surgical out-patient settings
Daily Self-Rating Scale for Depression (KUSTA)	Wendt *et al* (1985)	Self-rating	9	Assesses course of depressive illness
Newcastle scales	Carney *et al* (1965)	Physician rating	10	Used for differential diagnosis of endogenous and reactive depression
Montgomery–Åsberg Depression Rating Scale (MADRS)	Montgomery & Åsberg (1979)	Observer rating scale	17	Sensitive to change in depressive illness
Zung Self-Rating Depression Scale (SDS)	Zung (1965)	Self-rating	20	Can differentiate depression from other psychotic disorders
Carroll Depression Rating Scale	Carroll *et al* (1981)	Self-rating	17	Self-administered Hamilton scale

favour of assessment of behavioural symptoms and somatic complaints. They concluded on the basis of their own analysis that it was inferior to the Bech–Rafaelsen Melancholia Scale (BRMS) and the Montgomery–Åsberg Depression Rating Scale (MADRS) in respect of mean discriminating power, internal consistency, homogeneity and transferability. In general the

MADRS is more suitable in the presence of physical disorders with an enhanced somatic element. (A more detailed review of the HRDS is provided by Hedlund & Vieweg (1979).)

The self-rating Beck Depression Inventory (BDI) was developed as an instrument to measure the depth of depression (Beck *et al*, 1961). The items were clinically derived following systematic observation of depressed patients. Each of the 21 categories describes a series of four statements assigned values from 0 to 3 to indicate the level of severity, although some items are given an identical rating. The schedule was originally read out to the patient by a trained interviewer who chose the most appropriate statement in each category reflecting the patient's attitudes at the time of interview. The patient also has a copy of the interview to read and the scoring system obviously takes into account the number of symptoms in addition to their severity. The inventory has been found to parallel changes in the clinical assessment of severity of depressive disorder (Beck & Beamesderfer, 1974). Traditionally, however, the BDI has been considered to be subject to halo effects and therefore could not be depended on when assessing treatment outcome. A survey based on meta-analysis procedures by Edwards *et al* (1984) paradoxically found that the BDI is significantly less liberal than the HRSD. It has also been suggested that both the BDI and the Carroll Self-Rating Scale primarily measure a social undesirability response set in view of the fact that they both correlate as highly with social undesirability as with each other (Langevin & Stancer, 1979). More recently criticism of the BDI has centred around its performance when compared with other scales. Kearns *et al* (1982) suggest that the BDI and the Zigmond & Snaith (1983) inventory should now be abandoned in research, although this view is not universally held.

The CES–D scale is a short, structured, self-report scale designed to measure depressive symptoms in epidemiological studies (Radloff, 1977). Its components include depressed mood, feelings of guilt and worthlessness, feelings of helplessness and hopelessness, psychomotor retardation, loss of appetite, and sleep disturbance, all of which are rated over the previous week. Individual symptoms are scored from 0 to 3 with a total score range of 0–60. Most of the items are negatively worded, although for four of them this procedure is reversed in order to prevent a particular response set. The CES–D has been found to be reasonably good at screening out non-depressed subjects but in one study it correctly indentified only 60% of subjects who were considered to suffer from major depression according to the RDC and 71% of subjects with minor depression (Roberts & Vernon, 1983). In view of the modest agreement with RDC diagnoses in a community setting, the CES–D would seem to be most appropriate as an initial screening instrument.

Because so many depression scales include various manifestations of physical disorder, they are frequently of limited use in the setting of a medical or surgical out-patient department. The Zung Self-Rating Depression Scale, for example, is liable to miss those who present under the guise of somatic illness (Raft *et al*, 1977). Zigmond & Snaith (1983) therefore excluded symptoms of somatic reference and developed a 14-item scale for detecting the two most common disorders of anxiety and depression in a medical out-patient setting. Each item is scored 0–3 depending on severity. The cut-off point in either subscale of seven items can be set according to the requirement of the research project (e.g. low proportion of false positives: 10–11; low proportion of false negatives: 8–9). They also found that the scale is a valid measure of severity and can therefore be used to assess changes in mental state over time, in addition to its use as a screening instrument.

Rating scales for obsessive–compulsive symptoms

Hodgson & Rachman (1977) developed the Maudsley Obsessional–Compulsive Inventory (MOCI) to measure obsessional symptoms associated with observable rituals. The subject gives a true/false reply to a series of 30 questions which are organised in such a way as to prevent an obsessional acquiescent response set. The authors identified four subscales of symptoms, the principal two being checking and cleaning in addition to slowness and doubting. The inventory is not diagnostic (other diagnostic schedules, e.g. SCID, may be used for this purpose – see above) but attempts to differentiate between symptoms and obsessional personality traits. The MOCI scale is short and easy to administer.

The Leyton Obsessional Inventory on the other hand is a longer and more cumbersome instrument of 69 questions with yes/no answers (Cooper, 1970). It utilises a supervised card-sorting technique and both present obsessional symptoms and personality traits are measured. It is not corrected for an obsessional response set but can be administered by a non-medically qualified interviewer. Its original purpose was to assist in the assessment of house-proud women in a community survey, and it provides for both an indication of the range of obsessional symptoms present and the degree of resistance and interference associated with each symptom. Not unexpectedly, with such instruments the more obsessional patients take a considerable time to complete it. Robertson & Mulhall (1979) have developed a matrix scoring method which enhances the quality of the information obtained.

Obsessional symptoms can also be rated by other, more general instruments including the self-rating Middlesex Hospital Questionnaire (Crown & Crisp, 1966) and the Hopkins Symptom Checklist (Frank *et al*, 1957). The observer-rated CPRS has been used to generate an obsessional subscale of six items: compulsive thoughts, phobia, indecision, worrying over trifles, rituals, and inner tension; it is sensitive to change during the course of treatment and can be used in outcome studies of obsessional illness.

Anxiety scales

The selection of anxiety scales (see Table 9.6) inevitably depends on the clinical population to be assessed. Most of the observer-rated scales are

TABLE 9.6
Anxiety scales

Name	Author	No. of items	Main features
Hamilton Rating Scale for Anxiety	Hamilton (1959)	96	Scored at a clinical interview Used to measure response to treatment
Zung Anxiety Scale	Zung (1971)	20	Clinical scale based on observed behaviour and patient replies
Manifest Anxiety Scale	Freeman (1953)	56	Unique projective test Questionnaire filled in by subject
Stimulus Response Inventory	Endler *et al* (1962)	14 (11)	Differentiates anxiety responses from anxiety-producing situations Self-rating
Manifest Anxiety Scale	Taylor (1953)	50	Differentiates situational from non-situational anxiety Self-rating
Affect Adjective Checklist	Zucherman & Lubin (1965)	21	Distinguishes trait from state anxiety Self-report
Clinical Anxiety Scale	Snaith *et al* (1982)	6	Derived from Hamilton scale and based on clinical interview
Buss Rating Scale	Buss (1955)	20	Assessment by clinical interview
Anxiety Scale	Covi *et al* (1981), and see Lipman (1982)	26	5-point scale Assesses anxiety on basis of verbal report, behaviour and somatic symptoms

designed for use with psychiatric patients and are not appropriate for use in situational anxiety where self-rating scales have been more commonly used (e.g. with patients about to undergo a surgical procedure).

The Hamilton Rating Scale for Anxiety (HRSA; Hamilton, 1959) has not achieved the same prominence as its depression counterpart, but has nonetheless been in reliable use for many years. The 14 sections that are somatically biased cover the whole range of anxiety neurosis and are rated during a course of an unstructured interview after which additional information is sought if any specific ratings remain unclear. It has been extensively used as a measure of change in treatment outcome studies and its ratings of 0–4 are based on both subject replies and observed behaviour during the interview.

As mentioned earlier, the HADS can be used to measure anxiety in a medical out-patient setting where there is an additional need to take into account the influence of somatic symptoms. The Brief Scale for Anxiety (Tyrer *et al*, 1984) is another derivative of the CPRS and comprises ten items, all of which are rated on a seven-point scale. It can be used for assessing pathological anxiety on its own or in the presence of mixed states with depressive, phobic, obsessional or psychotic symptoms.

Snaith *et al* (1982) carried out an item analysis of the Hamilton scales and found that six symptoms were sufficient for rating anxiety over the previous two days. The items include psychic tension, muscular tension, hyperarousability, worrying, apprehension, and restlessness, and are provided with clear scoring instructions in the Clinical Anxiety Scale (Snaith *et al*, 1982).

Anxiety rating scales have been developed for other, more specific purposes, including drug withdrawal programmes (Merz & Ballmer, 1983) and in assessing level of sexual anxiety (Patterson & O'Gorman, 1986).

Psychogeriatric rating scales

The use of rating scales in the elderly (Table 9.7) brings special problems in view of the likely mix of physical and psychiatric pathology. Scales used in younger age groups are not usually sensitive to change in cognitive function and rarely cover the full range of symptoms required to assess treatment effects in elderly demented patients. Because of the present state of pharmacotherapy in old age there is a need to evaluate small and subtle changes in mental state in this age bracket. However, standard scales and inventories may be equally appropriate, depending on the circumstances, for example, the use of the HRSD and the CPRS in non-organic states. A brief discussion of available rating scales follows but it is not proposed to review psychometric tests for cognitive function.

One of the most widely used scales in the area of pharmacological research in senile dementia has been the Sandoz Clinical Assessment Geriatric Scale (Shader *et al*, 1974). A manual has been prepared (Venn, 1983) that provides detailed instructions on how to score each symptom on a seven-point scale. The five-factor structure has been substantiated by cross-cultural studies and has been found to discriminate between different levels of cognitive functioning. Because of the subjective nature of many of the items, it is recommended that it be supported by appropriate psychometric and neurophysiological tests wherever possible. Despite the inevitable problems that might be associated with a self-assessment scale in demented patients, one such scale has been developed (Yesavage *et al*, 1981). Because of the problem of reliability and validity it may best function as a screening instrument. A detailed evaluation of ward behaviour rating scales for psychogeriatric use is provided by Honigfeld (1981).

The Short-Care (Gurland *et al*, 1984) is a semistructured interview in two parts, the first of which examines symptoms of depression, dementia, subjective memory impairment, sleep disturbance, somatic symptoms and disability. The second part provides for operational diagnoses termed 'pervasive depression', 'pervasive dementia' and 'personal time dependency' (the amount of someone else's personal time required by the patient in order

TABLE 9.7
Psychogeriatric rating scales

Name	Authors	Main features
London Psychogeriatric Rating Scale	Hirsch *et al* (1978)	Global assessment of patient's level of functioning including mental status 36 items, each scoring 0–2 4 subscales: mental disability, sociality, irritating behaviour, and disengagement
Geriatric Behavioural Self-Assessment Scale	Yesavage *et al* (1981)	Self-rating modelled after SCAG (see below) Limited to less disturbed patients–mild to moderate dementia 18 items
Sandoz Clinical Assessment Geriatric Scale (SCAG)	Venn (1983), Shader *et al* (1974)	18 items, observer-rated Covers: cognitive function, mood and behaviour, daily living coping abilities, somatic complaints and global assessment of response to treatment
Stockton Geriatric Rating Scale	Meer & Baker (1966)	Original version has 33 items British version reduced to 18 (Gilliard & Pattie, 1977) Covers: physical disability, apathy communication difficulties and social disturbance
Short-Care	Gurland *et al* (1984)	Derived from the Comprehensive Assessment and Referral Evaluation (CARE) (Gurland *et al*, 1977) Covers: depression, dementia and disability Semistructured interview
Clinical Rating Scale for Symptoms of Psychosis in Alzheimer's Disease (SPAD)	Reisberg & Ferris (1985)	5 items, observer-rated, 0–3 Covers: specific types of delusion and purposeless activity For the assessment of antipsychotic drugs in Alzheimer's disease
Physical and Mental Impairment of Function Evaluation (PAMIE)	Gurel *et al* (1972)	Assesses psychiatric and physical status in addition to self-care and social function on the basis of ward behaviour

to cope), which are comparable to standard diagnoses only insofar as they could indicate the need for further investigation or treatment. The scale can be applied by non-psychiatrists and may be used as a screening instrument in community populations.

Other, more specific rating scales have been developed for individual conditions, including Alzheimer's disease (Reisberg & Ferris, 1985). The authors felt that existing scales did not cover the particular types of perceptual and thought disturbances experienced by Alzheimer patients and therefore described a simple five-item scale to cover these symptoms.

Personality disorder

A number of instruments specifically designed to diagnose personality disorders have become available during the past ten years. In this area of research more than any other it is usually necessary to get information from an objective source, but only some of the schedules listed in Table 9.8 are capable of doing this. In general, diagnosis is best made using structured interview schedules that can be augmented with subjective questionnaire data if required. Classification of personality disorders does not, as yet, command universal acceptance and the instrument chosen may yield either DSM–III–R or ICD–10 (draft) (World Health Organization, 1987) diagnoses. An alternative approach using the Personality Assessment Schedule (PAS; Tyrer & Alexander, 1979) yields five main personality categories (normal, schizoid, passive, dependent, anankastic and sociopathic) with a further nine subcategories if required. This instrument, which was empirically derived, is sufficiently flexible to give dimensional personality trait scores in addition to the diagnostic categories listed above and has

TABLE 9.8
Instruments for assessing personality disorder

Structured interview	Authors	Main features
Structured Clinical Interview for DSM–III–R Personality Disorders (SCID II)	Spitzer & Williams (1987)	Yields DSM–III–R diagnoses Has had limited application so far Normally preceded by personality questionnaire Subject version only
Personality Assessment Schedule (PAS)	Tyrer & Alexander (1979)	Yields 5 diagnostic categories: sociopathic, schizoid, passive dependent, anankastic, and normal 9 subcategories in addition to DSM–III–R and ICD–10 equivalent Also yields dimensional personality trait scores Subject and informant versions
Standardised Assessment of Personality (SAP)	Mann *et al* (1981)	Revised version (via author) yields ICD–10 diagnosis plus 2 other categories (anxious, self-conscious) Informant version only
Personality Disorder Examination (PDE)	Loranger *et al* (1985)	Present version yields DSM–III–R diagnosis In early stages of development Subject version only Takes up to 2 hours to complete
Structured Interview for DSM–III Personality Disorders (SIDP)	Stangl *et al* (1985)	Yields DSM–III–R diagnoses Utilises information from subject and informant Measures personality attributes of past 5 years where change has occurred

Adapted from Ferguson & Tyrer (in press).

been used in a wide variety of patient groups in different cultural settings. A computerised package is available and can be used to derive ICD-10 (draft) and DSM–III–R equivalents, although it is not capable of putting into effect the strict operational criteria of the latter.

Global rating scales

These measurements are based on an overall numerical assessment of the patient's clinical state as judged by the investigator over a fixed time span and may refer to one particular component of mental state (e.g. mood) or the overall level of illness. Examples of visual analogue scales of this genre are those discussed by Aitken (1969) and Luria (1975).

Section D. Constructing a new rating instrument

If an extensive review of the literature shows that there is no measuring instrument available for the phenomenon being tested, it *may* be necessary to construct a rating scale specifically for the purpose of the study. This decision should not be made without considerable thought. Although it may seem fairly easy to design a new scale, it takes a great deal of time and trouble to test it adequately and if the instrument is never used again it would be extremely difficult for future investigators to make any comparison between studies. It is suggested that any investigators finding themselves in the position of thinking about constructing a new rating instrument should carefully examine Chapter 8. It is essential for the instrument to be tested with regard to reliability and, despite the intrinsic difficulties, some measure of validity is often also possible. For example, the assessment of incest is extremely difficult because of the sensitivity of the subject, but if a new instrument was designed to test this in an epidemiological survey it would be reasonable to test this beforehand on a population already known to have experienced incest and a control group of patients in whom incestuous contact has not occurred. Although the additional information derived from these populations is not confirmatory it would be pointless to go ahead with the instrument if the two populations scored similarly on the main items.

   If a new instrument is being constructed the investigator will have to decide whether a dimensional scale or a categorical one would be most appropriate. This depends on the nature of the subject being studied, but the personal predilection of the investigator also seems to play a major part. If a categorical scale is chosen each score must be defined clearly and not merely given a number. If a dimensional scale is chosen the assumption is usually made for statistical purposes that the intervals between each pair of consecutive points are the same for all parts of the scale. This may not be true (or more frequently is never tested) and some investigators have preferred to use scales in which there are no anchor points at all. The visual analogue scale (VAS), a

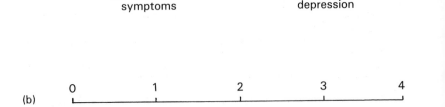

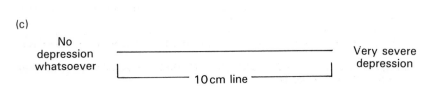

(c)

No depression whatsoever ――――――――――――――― Very severe depression
―――――― 10 cm line ――――――

Fig. 9.2   Examples of types of rating scale: (a) categorical scale, (b) interval scale (implying dimensions) ('Likert scales', see under 'Rating scale' in Glossary), (c) visual analogue scale – the subject is asked to place a vertical mark across the line at the point which best describes current feelings. This is then measured from the left-hand point to give the 'depression score'

somewhat pompous term to describe a linear scale with no anchor points, was popularised some years ago by Aitken (1969) and is often used in studies in which repeated measures are necessary because the scale is so easy to complete and is apparently sensitive to change. An example of the three types of scale using a common psychiatric symptom, depression, are illustrated in Fig. 9.2.

Although there is no clear-cut advice that can be given to the investigator as to which type of scale is superior, there is some evidence that better reliability is achieved when the number of scale points is seven or more (Cicchetti *et al*, 1985). It is preferable to have statistical advice before deciding on which approach to use.

References

ABRAMS, R. & TAYLOR, M. A. (1978) A rating scale for emotional blunting. *Amercian Journal of Psychiatry*, **135**, 226–229.
AITKEN, R. C. B. (1969) Measurement of feelings using visual analogue scales. *Proceedings of the Royal Society of Medicine*, **62**, 989–996.
AMERICAN PSYCHIATRIC ASSOCIATION (1980) *Diagnostic and Statistical Manual of Mental Disorders* (3rd edn) (DSM–III). Washington, DC: APA.

—— (1987) *Diagnostic and Statistical Manual of Mental Disorders* (3rd edn, revised) (DSM-III-R). Washington, DC: APA

ANDREASEN, N. C. (1979) Affective flattening and the criteria for schizophrenia. *American Journal of Psychiatry*, **136**, 944–947.

—— (1982) Negative symptoms in schizophrenia. *Archives of General Psychiatry*, **39**, 784–788.

ANGST, J., BATTEGAY, R., BENTE, D., *et al* (1967) Übern das gemeinsame vorgehen einer deutschen und schweizerchen Arbeitsgruppe auf den Gebiete der Psychiatrischen Dokumentation. *Schweizer Archiv für Neurologie Neurochirurgica und Psychiatrie*, **100**, 207–211.

ANTHONY, J., FOLSTEIN, M., ROMANOSKI, A., *et al* (1985) Comparison of the lay diagnostic interview schedule and a standardised psychiatric diagnosis. *Archives of General Psychiatry*, **42**, 667–675.

ÅSBERG, M., MONTGOMERY, S., PERRIS, C., *et al* (1978) The Comprehensive Psychopathological Rating Scale. *Acta Psychiatrica Scandinavica*, **271** (suppl. 5).

BECH, P. (1984) The instrumental use of rating scales for depression. *Pharmaco-Psychiatry*, **17**, 22–28.

——, BOLWIG, T. G., DEIN, E., *et al* (1975) Quantitative rating of manic states. *Acta Psychiatrica Scandinavica*, **52**, 1–6.

——, ——, KRAMP, P., *et al* (1979) The Bech–Rafaelsen Mania Scale and the Hamilton Depression Scale. *Acta Psychiatrica Scandinavica*, **59**, 420–430.

BECH, A. T., WARD, C. H., MENDELSON, M., *et al* (1961) An inventory for measuring depression. *Archives of General Psychiatry*, **4**, 561–571.

—— & BEAMESDERFER, A. (1974) Assessment of depression: the depressive inventory. Psychological measurements in psychopharmacology. *Modern Problems of Pharmacopsychiatry*, **7**, 151–169.

BEIGEL, A., MURPHY, D. L. & BUNNEY, W. E. (1971) The Manic State Rating Scale. *Archives of General Psychiatry*, **25**, 256–262.

BLACKBURN, J. M., LONDON, J. B. & ASHWORTH, C. M. (1977) A new scale for measuring mania. *Psychological Medicine*, **7**, 453–458.

BUSS, A., WEINER, M., DURKER, A., *et al* (1955) The measurement of anxiety in the clinical situation. *Journal of Consulting and Clinical Psychology*, **19**, 125–129.

CARNEY, M. W. P., ROTH, M. & GARSIDE, R. F. (1965) The diagnosis of depressive syndromes and the prediction of ECT response. *British Journal of Psychiatry*, **111**, 659–674.

CARROLL, B. J., FEINBERG, M. & SMOUSE, P. E. (1981) The Carroll Rating Scale for Depression 1. Development, reliability and validation. *British Journal of Psychiatry*, **138**, 194–200.

CICCHETTI, D. V., SHOWALTER, D. & TYRER, P. (1985) The effects of number rating scale categories on levels of inter-rater reliability: a Monte Carlo investigation. *Applied Psychological Measurement*, **9**, 31–36.

CLOUSTON, T. S. (1911) *Unsoundness of Mind.* London: Methuen.

COOPER, J. (1970) The Leyton Obsessional Inventory. *Psychological Medicine*, **1**, 48–64.

——, KENDALL, R. E., GURLAND, B. J., *et al* (1972) *Psychiatric Diagnosis in New York and London.* London: Oxford University Press.

COVI, L., RICKELS, K., LIPMAN, O. S., *et al* (1981) Effects of psychotropic agents on primary depression. *Psychopharmacology Bulletin*, **17**, 100–101.

CROWN, S. & CRISP, A. H. (1966) A short clinical dianostic self-rating scale for psychoneurotic patients. The Middlesex Hospital Questionnaire (MHQ). *British Journal of Psychiatry*, **112**, 917–923.

CSERNANSKY, J. G., YESAVAGE, J. A., MALONEY, W., *et al* (1983) The Treatment Response Scale: a retrospective method of assessing response to neuroleptics. *American Journal of Psychiatry*, **140**, 1210–1213.

EDWARDS, B., LAMBERT, M., MORAN, P., *et al* (1984) A meta analytic comparison of the Bech Depression Inventory and the Hamilton Rating Scale for Depression as measures of treatment outcome. *British Journal of Clinical Psychology*, **23**, 93–99.

ENDICOTT, J. & SPITZER, R. L. (1978) A diagnostic interview – the schedule for affective disorders and schizophrenia. *Archives of General Psychiatry*, **35**, 837–844.

ENDLER, N. S., HUNT, J. N. & ROSENSTEIN, A. J. (1962) The Stimulus Response Inventory. *Psychological Monograph*, **76**, 1–33.

FEIGHNER, J. P., ROBINS, E., GUZE, S. B., *et al* (1972) Diagnostic criteria for use in psychiatric research. *Archives of General Psychiatry*, **26**, 57–63.

FERGUSON, B. & TYRER, P. (1989) *Personality Disorder: Implements of Psychiatric Research*. London: John Wiley & Sons.

FOULDS, G. A. (1965) *Personality and Personal Illness*. London: Tavistock.

—— & HOPE, K. (1968) *Manual of the Symptom Sign Inventory (SSI)*. London: University of London Press.

FRANK, J. D., GLIEDMAN, L. H., IMBER, S. D., *et al* (1957) Why patients leave psychiatry. *AMA Archives of Neurology and Psychiatry*, **77**, 283–299.

FREEMAN, M. J. (1953) The development of a test for measurement of anxiety: a study of its reliability and validity. *Psychological Medicine Monograph Supplement*, **67**, 1–19.

GOLDBERG, D. (1972) *The Detection of Psychiatric Illness by Questionnaire*. Maudsley Monographs. London: Oxford University Press.

GRINGRAS, M. (1980) Validation of the General Practitioner Clinical Research Group 11 item depression scale. *Journal of International Medical Research*, **8**, (suppl. (3)45), 100.

GUREL, L., LINN, M. N. & LINN, B. S. (1972) Physical and mental impairment of function evaluation in the aged: the PAMIE Scale. *Journal of Gerontology*, **27**, 83–90.

GURLAND, B., KURIANSKY, J., SHARP, L., *et al* (1977–78) CARE: rationale, development and reliability. *International Journal of Aging and Human Development*, **8**, 9–42.

——, GOLDEN, R., TERESI, J., *et al* (1984) The Short-Care: an efficient instrument for the assessment of depression, dementia and disability. *Journal of Gerontology*, **39**, 166–169.

HAMILTON, M. (1959) The assessment of anxiety state by ratings. *British Journal of Medical Psychology*, **32**, 50–55.

—— (1960) A rating scale for depression. *Journal of Neurology, Neurosurgery and Psychiatry*, **23**, 56–62.

HEDLUND, J. & VIEWEG, B. W. (1979) The Hamilton Rating Scale for Depression – A comprehensive review. *Journal of Operational Psychiatry*, **10**, 149–165.

HEINRICHS, D. W., HANLON, T. E. & CARPENTER, W. T. (1984) The Quality of Life Scale: an instrument for rating the schizophrenic deficit syndrome. *Schizophrenia Bulletin*, **10**, 388–398.

HELZER, J. E., ROBINS, L. N., MCEVOY, L. T., *et al* (1985) A comparison of clinical and diagnostic interview schedule diagnoses. Physician re-examination of lay interviewed cases in the general population. *Archives of General Psychiatry*, **42**, 657–666.

HERSCH, E., KRAL, V. A. & BRUCE-PALMER, R. (1978) Clinical value of the London Psychogeriatric Rating Scale. *Journal of American Geriatric Society*, **26**, 348–354.

HESSELBROCK, V., STABENONE, J., HESSELBROCK, M., *et al* (1982) A comparison of two interview schedules. The Schedule for Affective Disorders and Schizophrenia Lifetime and the National Institute for Mental Health Diagnostic Interview Schedule. *Archives of General Psychiatry*, **39**, 674–677.

HODGSON, R. J. & RACHMAN, S. (1977) Obsessional compulsive complaints. *Behaviour Research and Therapy*, **15**, 389–395.

HONIGFELD, G. (1981) The evaluation of Ward Behaviour Rating Scales for psychogeriatric use. *Psychopharmacology Bulletin*, **17**, 82–95.

——, GILLIS, R. D. & KLELT, C. J. (1966) NOSIE-30: A treatment sensitive ward behaviour scale. *Psychological Reports*, **19**, 180–182.

IAGER, A. C., KIRCH, D. G. & WYATT, R. J. (1985) A negative symptom rating scale. *Psychiatry Research*, **16**, 27–36.

KEARNS, N. P., CRUICKSHANK, K., MCGUIGAN, K. J., *et al* (1982) Comparison of depression rating scales. *British Journal of Psychiatry*, **141**, 45–49.

KRAWIECKA, M., GOLDBERG, D. & VAUGHAN, M. (1977) A standardised psychiatric assessment scale for rating chronic psychotic patients. *Acta Psychiatrica Scandinavica*, **55**, 229–308.

LANGEVIN, R. & STANCER, H. (1979) Evidence that depression rating scales primarily measure a social undesirability response set. *Acta Psychiatrica Scandinavica*, **59**, 70–79.

LEIGHTON, D. C., HARDING, J. S., MACKLIN, D. C., *et al* (1963) *The Character of Danger*. New York: Basic Books.

LEWINE, R. R., FOGG, L. & MELTZER, H. Y. (1983) Assessment of negative and positive symptoms in schizophrenia. *Schizophrenia Bulletin*, **9**, 368–376.

LIPMAN, R. S., COLE, J. O., PARK, L. C., *et al* (1965) Sensitivity of symptom and non-symptom focused criteria of out-patient drug efficacy. *American Journal of Psychiatry*, **122**, 24–27.

LORANGER, A. W., SUSMAN, V. L., OLDHAM, J. M., *et al* (1985) *Personality Disorder Examination (PDE): a structured interview for DSM–III–R and ICD–9 personality disorders*. WHO/ADAMHA pilot version. White Plains, New York: The New York Hospital-Cornell Medical Center, Westchester Division.

LORR, M., KLELT, C. J., MCNAIR, D. M., *et al* (1963) In-patient Multidimensional Psychiatric Scale (Manual). Palo Alto: Consulting Psychological Press.

LURIA, R. E. (1975) The validity and reliability of a visual analogue mood scale. *Journal of Psychiatric Research*, **12**, 51–57.

—— & BERRY, R. (1979) Reliability and descriptive validity of PSE syndromes. *Archives of General Psychiatry*, **36**, 1187–1195.

MACMILLAN, A. M. (1957) The Health Opinion Survey: technique for estimating prevalence of psychoneurotic and related types of disorder in communities. *Psychological Reports*, **1**, 325–339.

MAIER, W. & PHILIPP, M. (1985) Comparative analysis of observer depression scales. *Acta Psychiatrica Scandinavica*, **72**, 239–245.

MANN, A. H., JENKINS, R., CUTTING, J. C., *et al* (1981) The development and use of a standardized assessment of abnormal personality. *Psychological Medicine*, **11**, 839–847.

MAURER, M., KIMY, S., WOGGON, B., *et al* (1984) Comparison of AMP System and the CPRS with regard to inter-rater reliability. *Neuropsychobiology*, **12**, 27–33.

MCMORDIE, W. & SWINT, E. (1979) Predictive utility, sex of rater differences and inter-rater reliabilities of the NOSIE 30. *Journal of Clinical Psychology*, **35**, 773–775.

MEER, B. & BAKER, I. A. (1966) The Stockton Geriatric Rating Scale. *Journal of Gerontology*, **21**, 393–403.

MERZ, W. A. & BALLMER, V. R. S. (1983) Symptoms of the barbiturate/benzodiazepine withdrawal syndrome in healthy volunteers: standardised assessment by a newly developed rating scale. *Journal of Psychoactive Drugs*, **15**, 71–84.

MILLER, I., BISHOP, S., NORMAN, W., *et al* (1985) The modified Hamilton Rating Scale for Depression: reliability and validity. *Psychiatry Research*, **14**, 131–142.

MONTGOMERY, S. A. & ÅSBERG, M. (1979) A new depression scale designed to be sensitive to change. *British Journal of Psychiatry*, **134**, 382–389.

—— & MONTGOMERY, D. B. (1980) Measurement of change in psychiatric illness, new obsessional, schizophrenia and depression scales. *Postgraduate Medical Journal*, **50** (suppl. I), 50–52.

NASR, S., ALTMAN, E., RODIN, M., *et al* (1984) Correlation of the Hamilton and Carroll Depression Rating Scales. A replication study among psychiatric out-patients. *Journal of Clinical Psychiatry*, **45**, 167–168.

OVERALL, J. E. (1974) The Brief Psychiatric Rating Scale in psychopharmacology research. Psychological measurements in psychopharmacology. *Modern Problems of Pharmacopsychiatry*, **7**, 67–68.

—— & GORHAM, D. R. (1962) The Brief psychiatric rating scale. *Psychological Reports*, **10**, 799–812.

—— & HOLLISTER, L. E. (1979) Compative evaluation of research diagnostic criteria for schizophrenia. *Archives of General Psychiatry*, **36**, 1198–1205.

PARLOFF, M. B., KELMAN, H. C. & FRANK, J. D. (1954) Comfort, effectiveness and self-awareness as criterion for improvement in psychotherapy. *American Journal of Psychiatry*, **111**, 343–351.

PATTERSON, D. G. & O'GORMAN, E. C. (1986) The SOMA – a questionnaire measure of sexual anxiety. *British Journal of Psychiatry*, **149**, 63–67.

PAYKEL, E. S. (1985) The Clinical Interview for Depression. Development, reliability and validity. *Journal of Affective Disorders*, **9**, 85–96.

PETTERSON, V., FYRO, B. & SEDVAL, C. (1973) A new scale for the longitudinal rating of manic states. *Acta Psychiatrica Scandinavica*, **49**, 248–256.

PLATMAN, S. R., PLUTCHIK, R., FIEVE, R. R., *et al* (1969) Emotion profiles associated with mania and depression. *Archives of General Psychiatry*, **20**, 210–214.

PLUTCHIK, R. (1967) The affective differential: emotion profiles implied by diagnostic concepts. *Psychological Reports*, **20**, 19–25.

RADLOFF, L. S. (1977) The CES–D scale: a self report depression scale for research in the general population. *Applied Psychological Measures*, **1**, 385–401.

RAFAELSEN, O. J., BECH, P., BOLWIG, T. G., *et al* (1980) The Bech–Rafaelsen combined rating scale for mania and melancholia. *Psychiatrica Fennica Supplementum*, 327–331.

RAFT, D., SPENCER, R., TOOMEY, T., *et al* (1977) Depression in medical out-patients: use of the Zung Scale. *Diseases of the Nervous System*, 999–1004.

REISBERG, B. & FERRIS, S. (1985) A clinical rating scale for symptoms of psychosis in Alzheimer's disease. *Psychopharmacology Bulletin*, **21**, 101–104.

RICKELS, K., GARCIA, C. R., LIPMAN, R., *et al* (1976) The Hopkins symptom checklist – assessing emotional distress in obstetric and gynaecological practice. *Primary Care*, **3**, 751–763.

ROBERTS, R. & VERNON, S. (1983) The Center for Epidemiologic Studies Depression Scale: its use in a community sample. *American Journal of Psychiatry*, **140**, 41–46.

ROBERTSON, J. R. & MULHALL, D. J. (1979) The clinical value of obsessionality: a development of the Leyton Obsessional Inventory. *Psychological Medicine*, **9**, 147–154.

ROBINS, L., HELZER, J., CROUGHAN, J., *et al* (1979) *The National Institute of Mental Health Diagnostic Interview Schedule*. Rockville: National Institute of Mental Health.

SHADER, R. I., HARMATZ, J. S. & SALZMAN, C. A. (1974) A new scale for clinical assessment of geriatric populations. Sandoz Clinical Assessment Geriatric (SCAG). *Journal of the American Geriatrics Society*, **22**, 107–113.

SHEPHERD, M., COOPER, B., BROWN, A. C., *et al* (1981) *Psychiatric Illness in General Practice*. New York: Oxford University Press.

SNAITH, R. P. (1981) Rating scales. *British Journal of Psychiatry*, **138**, 512–514.

——, BAUGH, S. J., CLAYDEN, A. D., *et al* (1982) The Clinical Anxiety Scale: an instrument derived from the Hamilton Anxiety Scale. *British Journal of Psychiatry*, **141**, 518–523.

SPIRO, H., SIASSI, I. & CROCETTI, G. (1972) What gets surveyed in a psychiatric survey? A case study of the MacMillan index. *Journal of Nervous and Mental Disease*, **154**, 105–114.

SPITZER, R. L., ENDICOTT, J. & ROBINS, E. (1975) Research Diagnostic Criteria (RDC). *Psychopharmacology Bulletin*, **11**, 22–24.

——, WILLIAMS, J. B. W. & GIBBON, M. (1985) *Instruction Manual for the Structured Clinical Interview for DSM–III–R (SCID, 7.1.85 revision)*. Biometrics Research Department. New York State Psychiatric Institute, 722 West 168th Street, New York, NY 10032.

—— & —— (1987) *Structured Clinical Interview for DSM–III–R Personality Disorders*. Biometrics Research Department, New York State Psychiatric Institute, 722 West 168th Street, New York, NY 10032.

STANGL, D., PFOHL, B., ZIMMERMAN, M., *et al* (1985) Structured interview for DSM–III personality disorders. *Archives of General Psychiatry*, **42**, 591–596.

TAYLOR, J. A. (1953) A personality scale of manifest anxiety. *Journal of Abnormal Social Psychology*, **48**, 285–290.

TSUANG, M. T. & WINOKUR, G. (1975) The Iowa 500: field work in a 35 year follow-up of depression, mania and schizophrenia. *Canadian Psychiatric Association Journal*, **20**, 359–365.

——, WOOLSTON, R. F. & SIMPSON, J. C. (1980) The Iowa Structured Psychiatric Interview. *Acta Psychiatrica Scandinavica*, **62**, (suppl. 283).

TYRER, P. & ALEXANDER, J. (1979) Classification of personality disorder. *British Journal of Psychiatry*, **135**, 163–167.

——, OWEN, R. T. & CICCHETTI, D. V. (1984) The Brief Scale for Anxiety: a subdivision of the Comprehensive Psychopathological Rating Scale. *Journal of Neurology, Neurosurgery and Psychiatry*, **47**, 970–975.

VAN DE HOUT, M. A. & GRIEZ, E. (1984) Validity and utility of the PSE in assessing neurosis: empirical findings and critical consideration. *Journal of Psychiatric Research*, **18**, 161–172.

VENN, R. D. (1983) The Sandoz Clinical Assessment – Geriatric Rating (SCAG) Scale. A general purpose psychogeriatric rating scale. *Gerontology*, **29**, 185–198.

WENDT, G., BINZ, V. & MÜLLER, A. A. (1985) KUSTA (Kurz-Skala Stimmung/Aktivierung): a daily self-rating scale for depressive patients. *Pharmacopsychiatry*, **18**, 118–122.

WING, J. K., COOPER, J. E. & SARTORIUS, N. (1974) *Measurement and Classification of Psychiatric Symptoms: an Instruction Manual for the PSE and Catego Program*. London: Cambridge University Press.

WORLD HEALTH ORGANIZATION (1973) *The International Pilot Study of Schizophrenia*. Geneva: WHO.

—— (1987) ICD-10. *Draft Version of Chapter V*. Geneva: WHO.

YESAVAGE, J., ADEY, M. & WERNER, P. (1981) Development of a geriatric behavioral self-assessment scale. *Journal of the American Geriatrics Society*, **29**, 285–288.

YOUNG, R. C., BIGGS, J. T., ZIEGLER, V. E., *et al* (1978) A rating scale for mania: reliability, validity and sensitivity. *British Journal of Psychiatry*, **133**, 429–435.

ZIGMOND, A. & SNAITH, R. (1983) The Hospital Anxiety and Depression Scale. *Acta Psychiatrica Scandinavica*, **67**, 361–370.

ZUCKERMAN, M. & LUBIN, B. (1965) *Manual for the Multiple Affect Adjective Checklist*. San Diego, California: Educational and Industrial Testing Service.

ZUNG, W. W. K. (1965) A self-rating depression scale. *Archives of General Psychiatry*, **12**, 63–70.

—— (1971) A rating instrument for anxiety disorders. *Psychosomatics*, **12**, 371–379.

10 Rating scales for special purposes. I: Psychotherapy

SIOBHAN MURPHY and PETER TYRER

This chapter addresses the problems of rating the more diffuse and difficult attributes that are often important in psychiatric practice. These are predominantly concerned with attitudes, behaviour and relationships. Unfortunately, although attempts have been made to develop a core battery of tests with general applicability (Waskow & Parloff, 1975) the validity of this approach has been questioned (Lambert *et al*, 1983). Nevertheless, the alternative has hardly been constructive. A recent review of 216 outcome studies published in the *Journal of Consulting and Clinical Psychology* between 1976 and 1980 revealed 254 different self-report measures alone (Lambert, 1983). Reviews of the available scales have been published (Waskow & Parloff, 1975; Hersen & Bellack, 1976; Lambert *et al*, 1983; Greenberg & Pinsoff, 1986) and this chapter discusses only general principles, and points the reader towards some of the more important scales in the field.

These scales are mainly used in evaluation of psychotherapy (Table 10.1) and, as psychotherapy is mainly concerned with intrapsychic change, it is not surprising that self-report measures are still the most popular type of

TABLE 10.1
Three critical dimensions of change in psychotherapy

Content	Process	Source
Intrapersonal	Judgemental (evaluational)	Self-report
Emotional	Descriptive	Therapist rating
Behavioural	Observational	Significant others
Cognitive	Physiological	Trained observer
Interpersonal		Institutional
Social role performance		

Adapted from Lambert *et al* (1986).

176

instrument (Lambert, 1983). The advantages and handicaps of self-report have been mentioned in Chapter 9, and they have also been discussed with regard to psychotherapy (Gynther & Green, 1982; Beutler & Crago, 1983).

Self-report measures

Although the Minnesota Multiphasic Personality Inventory (MMPI; Hathaway & McKinley, 1967) is primarily considered to be a measure of personality, it is a useful measure of attitudinal change and is still widely used despite criticisms (Gleser, 1975; Beutler & Crago, 1983). The inventory consists of 550 statements which are answered "True, False, or Cannot say". It yields 14 scores, 10 of which are clinical (hypochondriasis, depression, hysteria, psychopathic deviate, masculinity, femininity, paranoia, psychasthesia, schizophrenia, hypomania, social introversion) and four of which are validity scores (question, lie, validity, and correction). The 14 scores are used to plot profiles which are compared with standard scores. The interpretation of the profiles requires some skill and literal interpretation of the clinical scores is not advised. There are many psychometric reservations about the MMPI (Anastasi, 1968) but there is a huge comparative database and many widely used research scales have developed from it (e.g. the Barron Ego Strength Scale (Barron, 1953)). Beutler & Crago (1983) recommend it for demographic purposes but not as a measure of change.

Early studies of psychotherapy based primarily on Freudian theory made wide use of projective tests of personality (e.g. the Rorschach Inkblot Test (Klopfer, 1968) and the Thematic Apperception Test (TAT; Murray, 1943)). These fell out of favour in the 1960s and 1970s as they relied on subjective scoring, had poor psychometric data and were specific to theory. The scoring and administration of the Rorschach Inkblot Test has been standardised (Exner, 1978), improving its reliability, and its use as part of a battery has been suggested for child psychotherapy assessment (Tramontana & Sherrets, 1983).

The Hopkins Symptom Checklist (mentioned in Chapter 9) and its revised form (Derogatis *et al*, 1974; Lipman *et al*, 1979) are recommended by Waskow & Parloff (1975) and Beutler & Crago (1983) as a multisymptom checklist. The revised form (SCL–90–R) is a 90-item checklist rated on a five-point scale of distress, usually in the last week. It covers nine symptom dimensions and has three global indices of distress. Factor analysis (Lipman *et al*, 1979) yields eight factors: somatisation, phobic anxiety, retarded depression, agitated depression, obsessive–compulsive, interpersonal sensitivity, anger–hostility, and psychoticism. A wide range of norms from psychiatric and medical out-patients are available; it is sensitive to change and has good psychometric data.

Although many of these instruments are basically recording symptoms, they are popular in the assessment of psychotherapy because of their wide use and evidence that they are sensitive to change.

TABLE 10.2
Outcome measurements in psychotherapy: self-report scales

Name	Author	Main points
Hopkins Symptom Checklist HSCL–(58) SCL–(90)	Derogatis *et al* (1974) Lipman *et al* (1979)	Symptom inventories developed with out-patients; rated on 4-point (58) or 5-point (90) scale; yields 5(58) or 8(90) factors; takes 15 min to administer
Target Complaints[1]	Battle (1966)	Individualised scales based on usually 3 major complaints; variety of scoring methods; widely used as part of battery; not generalisable
Goal Attainment Scaling (GAS)[1]	Kiresuk & Sherman (1968)	Widely used individualised scale; goals set before treatment; scaled in terms of likely outcome; independent observer can rate; variable reliability; not generalisable
Minnesota Multiphasic Personality Inventory (MMPI)	Hathaway & McKinley (1967) Dahlstrom *et al* (1972)	Very widely used, controversial; 550 statements covering range of symptomatology, attitudes, demographic data; 14 scores yielded – profile developed; interpretation needs caution; multiple research scales
Butler–Haig Q Sort	Butler & Haig (1954)	Wide use; 100 statements on card yield measurement of self-concept
Impact of Event Scale	Horowitz *et al* (1979)	Stress-specific symptoms; 15-item scale; rated for frequency and intensity on 4-point scale; 2 subscales, intrusion and avoidance
Social Adjustment Scale Self-Report (SAS–S)	Weissman & Bothwell (1976)	Self-report form of Social Adjustment Scale; 42 items rated on 5-point scale, covering work, social, family, marital and economic roles

1. Can also be used as therapist measures.

Self-concept scales

Many studies have attempted to assess the concept of 'self', the most popular instruments being the Butler–Haig Q Sort (Butler & Haig, 1954) and the Personal Orientation Inventory (POI; Shostrom, 1966). The methodology of self-perception studies and scales available to measure self-perception are reviewed by Gordon (1969).

The Butler–Haig Q Sort consists of 100 statements printed on individual cards, reflecting personality traits and symptoms. These are sorted into piles according to instructions, usually 'most like me' and 'least like me'. The responses allow a self-ideal correlation (QSI) and a Q adjustment score (QAS) to be derived. These are sensitive to change and have satisfactory reliabilities. A defensiveness index allows scores to be adjusted for social desirability responses. Test–retest reliability is 0.76 for the QSI and 0.86 for the QAS. It takes a long time to complete.

The Personal Orientation Inventory is a questionnaire which yields 12 scores associated with self-realisation (e.g. self-regard, spontaneity, capacity for intimate contact). It is broader than the Butler–Haig Q Sort as it assesses more than the isolated concepts of 'ideal' and 'perceived' self. The reliability of the inventory varies between 0.55 and 0.85, which is reasonably good, but both the Personal Orientation Inventory and the Butler–Haig Q Sort were developed for client-centred therapies and may be too specific to theory. Briefer scales for measuring self-concept include the Personal Attribute Inventory (Kappes & Parish, 1979), the Rosenberg Self-Esteem Scale (Rosenberg, 1965) and its revision as the Self-Esteem Scale (O'Malley & Bachman, 1979). There is as yet no scale measuring change in self-control that has demonstrated usefulness as a measure of outcome, although the Rosenbaum (1980) Self-Control Schedule is an interesting development.

The recent interest in the DSM–III category 'post-traumatic stress disorder' (American Psychiatric Association, 1980) has led to the development of the Impact of Event Scale (Horowitz *et al*, 1979). This aims to assess the impact of recent severe life events rated on 15 items for frequency and intensity on a four-point scale. The characteristic qualities of intrusion and avoidance in post-traumatic stress disorder form separate subscales and a total stress score can be computed. Both subscales are sensitive to change, differentiate between populations and have satisfactory psychometric properties (Zilberg *et al*, 1982; Horowitz *et al*, 1986). Test–retest reliability for the total stress score is 0.87, for the intrusion subscale 0.89, and the avoidance subscale, 0.79.

The Social Adjustment Scale–Self-Report (SAS–SR; Weissman & Bothwell, 1976) is a written self-administered form of the Social Adjustment Scale (Weissman & Paykel, 1974). Its 42 questions measure affective and instrumental performance in occupational role, social and leisure activities, relationships with extended family, marital role, family unit and economic independence. It is quick to administer (15–20 minutes) and covers functioning in the last two weeks on a five-point scale. Role area mean scores and a total score are obtained. This is sensitive to change in depressed patients, is able to distinguish between groups, and has a range of available norms. The self-report overall score correlates ($r = 0.72$) with an observer's overall score on the Social Adjustment Scale (see below). This and other self-report scales are summarised in Table 10.2

Intrapsychic function

Most psychotherapy outcome studies include some measure of perceived improvement and overall satisfaction with treatment. While these measures have face validity, are easy to use and correlate well with other variables, they also have inherent difficulties. Few of the scales are standardised and they represent more the status of the patient at the end of the study than the change from status before therapy (Green *et al*, 1975; Garfield, 1978).

Beutler & Crago (1983) have suggested ways of improving these scales and offer a sample questionnaire. Patients are asked to rate their status (a) as they remember it to have been at the start of therapy and (b) as it is at the finish. The mean difference between the two scores is taken as the amount of treatment-related change. An index of patient-perceived improvement is obtained by combining global and specific change scores.

The development of individualised target complaints focusing on the specific problems bringing a patient to therapy has been fraught with difficulty (Kaltreider *et al*, 1981*a*). The most widely used techniques are the Target Complaints (Battle *et al*, 1966) and the Goal Attainment Scaling (GAS; Kiresuk & Sherman, 1978). The Target Complaints asks the patient at assessment to identify up to three principal complaints and rate them on a 13-point scale; these are then also rated at termination, either by the patient (Battle *et al*, 1966) or the therapist (Sloane *et al*, 1975). Target Complaints retains an attraction as a simple way of recording complaints which has face validity to the patient. It can offer additional information when it is used in conjunction with other outcome measures but its major limitations need to be borne in mind. The GAS is more refined, as a number of goals are set before treatment by the patient or between the patient and therapist. Each goal is scaled with a series of graded likely outcomes from the least to the most favourable. These can then be scored by an independent observer if required. A standard score can be derived. Problems with these measures include variable inter-rater agreement on setting and evaluation of goals (Calsyn & Davidson, 1978; Bond *et al*, 1979), the impossibility of comparisons across groups, and difficulty in assessing more complex dynamic change (rather than specific symptom change) as therapy progresses.

In an attempt to assess the more complex dynamic change involved in psychotherapy Malan (1963) proposed an individualised measure based on a formulation of "a basic neurotic conflict". The replication of the formulation approach has proved difficult (DeWitt *et al*, 1983) and is heavily dependent on trained clinicians. It has also been suggested that symptomatic improvement based on simple global measures comprised most of the observed change (Mintz, 1981).

The expert observer rater

Various scales for implementation by a trained observer are shown in Table 10.3. Waskow & Parloff (1975) recommended the use of the Psychiatric Status Schedule (PSS; Spitzer *et al*, 1970), which is a standardised interview aimed at the evaluation of psychopathology and role functioning. Its 321 items cover: mental state, role functioning, leisure activities, interpersonal relationship, and drug and alcohol abuse. These are judged as 'true' or 'false' over the last week or the last month for role functioning and drug and alcohol

TABLE 10.3
Trained observers scales

Name	Author	Main points
Psychiatric Status Schedule (PSS)[1]	Spitzer *et al* (1970)	Assesses psychopathology and role functioning; trained rater; standardised interview; 321 items; factor analysis yields 16 symptom scales and 6 role scales
Health Sickness Rating Scale (HSRS)[1]	Luborsky (1962)	Unitary and global ratings of mental health; range of scores 0–100 extends into normal functioning; interval scale with 8 descriptive anchors including behavioural and diagnostic criteria
Prognostic Index for Psychotherapy (PI)	Auerbach *et al* (1972)	Semistructured; lasts 60–90 min; 29 variables designed to predict outcome rated on 5-point scale
Global Assessment Scale (GAS)[1]	Endicott *et al* (1976)	Developed from HSRS (Luborsky, 1962); assesses overall functioning; scale 0–100 from illness–health; 10 descriptive anchors–only behavioural
Stress Response Rating Scale (SRRS)	Weiss *et al* (1984)	40 items; measures effect of severe life event; 3 subscales: intrusion, avoidance/denial, general stress; rated on 4-point scale
Social Adjustment Scale (SAS)	Weissman & Paykel (1974)	Derived from SSIAM (Gurland *et al*, 1972); trained rater; 41 items rated on 5-point scale; assesses role, role performance, role function and distress in 6 roles
Patterns of Individual Change Scales (PICS)	Kaltreider *et al* (1981)	Developed with bereaved patients; videotaped; 13 scales, 7 anchored points/scale; extends into 'normal' range of symptoms, social relationships and self-concept
Motivation for Psychotherapy Scale (MOPS)	Rosenbaum & Horowitz (1983)	23-item scale; 7-point scale; trained raters; 4 factors

1. Can also be used as therapist measures.

abuse. Factor analysis yields 17 symptom scales and six role scales. This scale was developed with in-patients and reported high reliability and sensitivity to change. When used to assess psychotherapy outcome in outpatients its sensitivity to change was lower (Strupp & Hadley, 1979). Other reservations about its use are discussed by Auerbach (1983). Observer rating scales with more emphasis on psychiatric diagnosis alone include the Schedule for Affective Disorders and Schizophrenia (SADS; Endicott & Spitzer, 1978), the Brief Psychiatric Rating Scale (BPRS; Overall & Gorham, 1962), the Present State Examination (PSE; Wing *et al*, 1974) and the Structured Clinical Interview for DSM–III (SCID; Spitzer *et al*, 1985) and are discussed in Chapter 9. The major advantage of the PSS is its broader view of a person's social functioning.

The Social Adjustment Scale (SAS; Weissman & Paykel, 1974) was derived from the Structured and Scaled Interview to Assess Maladjustment (SSIAM; Gurland *et al*, 1972). Its 41 questions focus on the same areas as the SAS–SR (see above) rating on a five-point scale, behaviour and feeling occurring over the last two and a half months. It is rather lengthy (45–90 minutes to complete). The SAS has good psychometric properties and is sensitive to change when used within the reference groups for which it was designed. It represents middle-class values and its validity outside these groups is questionable (Platt, 1981), and other scales are available that do not have the same preoccupation with social norms (Remington & Tyrer, 1979; Platt *et al*, 1980). Social Adjustment Scales have been extensively reviewed by Weissman (1975), and Weissman *et al* (1981).

The Stress Response Rating Scale (SRRS; Weiss *et al*, 1984) was developed, as was the Impact of Event Scale (Horowitz *et al*, 1979), to assess reaction to a recent, severe, life event. It consists of 40 items, 13 describing signs and symptoms of intrusion, 13 describing thought and behaviour indicative of avoidance and denial, and 14 describing general signs and symptoms of distress. It is rated on a four-point scale of severity over the last week. Inter-rater reliability of the intrusion scale ($r = 0.77$) and general stress scale ($r = 0.64$) are satisfactory, but reliability for the avoidance–denial subscale is rather low ($r = 0.43$). If pooled ratings are taken, the reliability level increases to 0.87, 0.78 and 0.60 respectively for the three scales. The SRRS is sensitive to change in bereaved patients following brief psychotherapy (Horowitz *et al*, 1984, 1986).

Global rating scales express change as the difference between global ratings made before and after therapy. The Health Sickness Rating Scale (HSRS; Luborsky, 1962) is a widely used example of a global scale. The patient's level of functioning is assessed on a 100-point scale which extends from total dependence to an ideal state of mental health. The assessment is made by considering: level of dependence/autonomy, severity of symptoms, level of discomfort and distress, effect on the environment, ability to utilise strengths, quality of relationships and depth of interests. In addition the global rating is made by comparison to a series of pre-rated clinical vignettes and nine anchor points describing behaviour and diagnostic criteria on the 100-point scale. The HSRS has satisfactory psychometric qualities and correlates with other clinical judgements.

The Global Assessment Scale (GAS; Endicott *et al*, 1976) was an attempt to simplify rating using the HSRS. It provides more anchor points, using only behavioural examples, and has discarded the clinical vignettes which had made the HSRS lengthy to score. Increased information is given about level of rating. The GAS is sensitive to change, has been used to predict rehospitalisation, correlates with other measures of illness and has an inter-rater reliability over five studies ranging from 0.69 to 0.91 (r).

The Patterns of Individual Change Scale (PICS; Kaltreider *et al*, 1981*b*) developed from attempts to provide individualised assessments, but instead of being tailored to the individual it is focused on populations. It was developed with a group of bereaved people, and allows cross-study comparisons to be made on dimensions of self-concept and interpersonal relationships while retaining the benefits of less generalised scales. It is based on video-rated assessments and consists of 13 scales with seven anchor points per scale. The scales extend into the normal range of functioning. The individual scales form a profile which can be used to assess patterns of change rather than change in specific symptoms. Initial analysis showed satisfactory inter-rater reliability (i.e. $r > 0.6$) on eight of the scales. Pooling observer ratings increases the reliability (Kalkreider *et al*, 1981*b*). The 13 scales are: grief, intrusion, avoidance, use of support, self-esteem, assertion, same-sex friendships, opposite-sex friendships, relation to siblings, children and surviving parent, work identity, and intimacy. Further psychometric data are presented by Weiss *et al* (1985).

The Prognostic Index for Psychotherapy (Auerbach *et al*, 1972) was developed to assess patients on variables believed to be of prognostic significance in psychotherapy, but it can also be used to assess change as some of its variables reflect emotional health. It is a 29-item semistructured interview covering demographic, past history and psychodynamic variables. Factor analysis yields five factors: level of adjustment, emotional freedom, aptitude for psychotherapy, acute depression, and intellectual freedom. Inter-rater reliability reflects the amount of training in using the schedule. This index is sensitive to change.

The issue of motivation for psychotherapy, partially reflected in the above factor 'aptitude for psychotherapy', has been very widely defined and has led to some confusion (Garfield, 1978). Rosenbaum & Horowitz (1983) attempted to tighten the concept of motivation in the Motivation for Psychotherapy Scale (MOPS). This is a 23-item scale rating video-taped interviews on a seven-point scale. Factor analysis yields four factors: active engagement, psychological mindedness, incentive-mediated willingness to sacrifice, and positive valuation of therapy. The concept of active engagement correlates most highly with global ratings ($r = 0.88$). While this scale is still being developed, it represents a needed attempt to standardise the ratings of the multifactorial concept of motivation.

Significant-others rating scales

These scales are summarised in Table 10.4. Strupp & Hadley's (1977) "tripartite model of mental health" emphasises the importance of using not only the patient and mental health workers as means of assessing mental health and change, but also significant others in the patient's life. While there are potential problems with this approach (Davidson & Davidson, 1983), it forms an essential part of a broad view of the effect of psychotherapy.

The two most widely used scales are the Katz Adjustment Scale – Relatives Form (KAS–R; Katz & Lyerly, 1963) and the Personal Adjustment and Role Skills Scale (PARS III; Ellsworth, 1975).

TABLE 10.4
Significant-others scales

Name	Author	Main points
Katz Adjustment Scale–Relatives Form (KAS–R)	Katz & Lyerly (1963)	205 items in 5 scales covering recent symptoms and behaviour, level of performance, respondents' expectations and satisfaction with performance; lengthy; pooled informant reliability; widely used
Personal Adjustment and Role Skills–III (PARS–III)	Ellsworth (1975)	Can be completed as postal questionnaire; widely used; shorter than KAS–R; separate male/female forms; 118 and 120 items; measures personal adjustment, role skills, drug/alcohol abuse
Social Behaviour Assessment Schedule (SBAS)	Platt *et al* (1980)	Evaluates change on patient and family due to medical/psychiatric illness; semistructured interview; trained rater; 239 items, 6 sections; takes 60–90 min; ratings defined; good psychometric data
Psychological Adjustment to Illness Scale (PAIS)	Derogatis (1976)	Rates adjustment to medical illness; semi-structured interview; trained rater; 45 questions assess functioning in 7 areas; rated on 4-point scale; takes 20–30 min; good psychometric data except for extended family relationships

The KAS–R contains five scales. The first, R_1, is a 127-item scale covering current psychiatric symptoms and social behaviour. This yields 13 clusters (belligerence, verbal expansiveness, negativism, helplessness, suspiciousness, anxiety, withdrawal and retardation, general psychopathology, nervousness, bizarreness, hyperactivity, and stability) and three factors: social obstreperousness, acute psychoticism, and withdrawal helplessness. R_2 is a 16-item scale describing level of performance of socially expected activities. R_3 has 16 items looking at a respondent's level of expectation for the patient's performance in these activities. R_4 has 23 items assessing free-time activities, and R_5 23 items assessing the respondent's satisfaction with the level of free-time activities. All the items are rated on a four-point Likert-type scale (see Chapter 9, p. 170). The whole scale takes between 30 and 60 minutes to complete. Discrepancy measures indicative of dissatisfaction with role performance and separate scale scores for R_1 to R_5 can be calculated. The KAS–R has been extensively developed and used. It has generated large amounts of normative, reliability and validity data and is sensitive to change (Fiske, 1975). Inter-rater reliability is high on scales judging observable behaviour (e.g. performance of socially expected activities) $(r = 0.85)$, and, as would be expected, low on scales judging informants' attitudes $(r = 0.28)$ (Crook *et al*, 1980).

The most recent version of PARS (PARS III; Ellsworth, 1975) was developed with a sample from a community clinic and gives separate scales for men and women which may be used as postal questionnaires. The 118-item male scale yields seven factors, four personal adjustment factors (interpersonal involvement, confusion, anxiety, agitation/depression) and one alcohol/drug factor, with two role skills factors – employment and outside social activities. The 120-item female version yields three personal adjustment factors (interpersonal involvement, confusion, agitation), one alcohol/drug factor, and two role skill factors – household management and outside social activities. There are two optional role factors, employment and parenthood skills. A household management and parenthood skills score has also been included in the male version. PARS scales also have large amounts of psychometric data available and have been extensively developed and reviewed (Fiske, 1975). Internal consistencies range from 0.77 to 0.98 and test–retest reliabilities from 0.74 to 0.98.

Many other scales have been used to obtain information from significant others (Fiske, 1975; Davidson & Davidson, 1983) but usually via an interviewer who scores the scales, thus introducing another level of bias. These scales include the Psychological Adjustment to Illness Scale (PAIS; Derogatis, 1976) and the Social Behaviour Assessment Schedule (SBAS; Platt *et al*, 1980) which have both been developed for use with medical patients. The SBAS has also been used with psychiatric patients and pays particular emphasis to the effect on the family, including an assessment of the informant's attitude towards the patient.

The Structured and Scaled Interview to Assess Maladjustment (SSIAM; Gurland *et al*, 1972) and the Social Adjustment Self-Report Scale (SAS–SR; Weissman & Bothwell, 1976) have also been used with significant others via an interviewer. The Social Adjustment Scale–II (SAS–II; Glazer *et al*, 1980) is a revision of the SAS–SR designed for schizophrenic patients. It rates eight areas: work as housewife, student or wage earner, relationship with principal household member, parental role, relationship with external family, social and leisure activities, conjugal and non-conjugal hetero-sexual behaviour, romantic involvement, and personal well-being. Both the SAS–II and the SAS–SR have shown high levels of agreement between patient and informant (Weissman & Bothwell, 1976; Glazer *et al*, 1980).

Therapist scales

The use of the therapist as rater of change has caused some debate (Lorr, 1975; Strupp & Bloxom, 1975; Mintz, 1977; Newman, 1983). The central issue has been the ability of the therapist to be objective about his/her own patients. Mintz *et al* (1973) found that the degree of unreliable reporting was similar for therapists, expert raters and clients, and suggest that the therapist is no better and no worse than any other rater and also offers a valuable alternative perspective.

A number of the scales reviewed above have also been used as therapist measures. These include the GAS (Endicott *et al*, 1976), the Goal Attainment Scaling (Kiresuk & Sherman, 1968), the BPRS (Overall & Gorham, 1962), the Psychiatric Status Schedule (Spitzer *et al*, 1970), and Target Complaints (Battle *et al*, 1966). Target Complaints is the only measure recommended by Waskow & Parloff (1975), although in their individual reviews Strupp & Bloxon (1975) also recommend the Rating Scales for Outcome of Therapy (Storrow, 1960), and Lorr (1975) recommends the Therapist Change Report (Lorr *et al*, 1962) and the Interpersonal Behaviour Inventory (IBI; Lorr & McNair, 1965).

The Rating Scales for Outcome of Therapy (Storrow, 1960) were developed to reflect areas of change in analytic psychotherapy. They are composed of 11 items covering five areas: symptoms and problems, productiveness, sexual adjustment, interpersonal relationships, and ability to handle stress. Single-scale scores are averaged for each area and summed to give a total outcome score. Inter-rater reliability is reported for therapist, expert observer, patient and relative. All correlations are above 0.5 with the exception of relative and therapist ($r = 0.32$), for whom levels of agreement are not very good.

The IBI consists of 140 behavioural statements rated on a four-point scale of frequency, covering 15 characteristic styles of interpersonal relationships. Factor analysis yields the following dimensions: dominance, competitiveness, aggression, mistrust, detachment, inhibition, submissiveness, succourence, abasement, deference, agreeableness, nurturance, affection, sociability, dependency, and hostility. Analysis of the total scores yields higher-level dimensions: control, nurturance, sociability, dependency, and hostility. Norms are available for psychiatric out-patients and normal controls. Internal consistency is high but no data are available for re-rating reliability.

The Therapist Change Report (Lorr *et al*, 1962) in a similar way to the Storrow scales, were developed to measure behavioural change expected in psychotherapy. Factor analysis yields five change factors: reduced physical complaints, reduced anxiety/depression, reduced hostility/agression, increased affection and acceptance of others and increased sociability. The scale is internally consistent and has been shown to be sensitive to change.

Process scales

The above scales have been used to study the effect of psychotherapy rather than what actually occurs within the session, as well as the therapist's and patient's views of the therapy. There have been many reviews of the process of psychotherapy and the many variables which contribute to this (Gurman & Razin, 1977; Rice & Greenberg, 1984; Greenberg & Pinsoff, 1986). It

TABLE 10.5
Process measures in psychotherapy

Name	Author	Main points
Relationship Inventory (RI)	Barret-Lennard (1962)	Therapist ± patient questionnaire; client-centred therapy; 85 items scored from – 3 to + 3; 5 variables; widely used
Accurate Empathy Scale (1)	Truax & Carkhuff (1967)	Used with observation ± tapes; 9 stages of scale evaluating therapist perception of client's feelings;
Unconditional Positive Regard Scale (2)		5 stages of scale measuring therapist warmth
Therapist Genuineness Scale (3)		5 stages of scale measuring genuineness; widely used; recent queries about replicability and validity (Mitchell *et al*, 1977)
Therapy Session Report (therapists' form) (patient form available) (TSR)	Orlinsky & Howard (1966)	Structured response questionnaire; 152 items; 3- or 4-point scale covers 10 facets of therapist's experience of self and patient
Vanderbilt Psychotherapy Process Scale (VPPS)	Gomes-Schwartz & Schwartz (1978)	Based on TSR; 84 items; video/audio recording for rating therapist's and patient's attitudes and behaviours; 8 factors; 5-point scale
Vanderbilt Negative Indicators Scale (VNIS)	Strupp *et al* (1981, unpublished)	Audio/visual recordings; trained raters; 42 items; 5 subscales rating patient and therapist activity; 6-point scale
Therapeutic Alliance Scale	Marziali *et al* (1981)	Used with audio-recorded sessions; 42-item scale, 21 therapist, 21 patient items; positive and negative items; 6-point scale of 'intensity of presence'; trained raters; 2 subscales
Therapist Action Scale (TAS) Patient Action Scale (PAS)	Hoyt *et al* (1981)	24 TAS, 25 PAS items; directed at activity in the session; audio recordings; trained raters; scored 0–5
Patient Experiencing Scale (short form) (EXP)	Klein *et al* (1969)	Audio rated; 7-point anchored annotated scale; clinically naive; judges degree of being in touch with immediate feelings
Therapist Experiencing Scale	Klein & Mathieu-Coughlan (1984)	Audio rated; 7-point anchored scale as above; concerned with therapist's focus on patient's words and therapist's manner
Counsellor Verbal Response Category System	Hill (1978)	Therapist's verbal behaviour rated; 14 categories; response units judged and categorised by independent trained judges
Modified Helper Behaviour Rating System	Shapiro *et al* (1984)	Modified from Elliot (1979) manual; 12 categories of verbal response; modified to include 'shared frame of reference'; trained raters of response units

is not possible to cover here all the variables that have been studied, but a variety of rating scales (Table 10.5), many specifically developed to study brief focal therapy, is examined to give an overview.

The choice of scales to use in process research depends upon the perspective of observation and the level of analysis wished to be studied (Elliott, 1984). Observations can be taken from the patient and therapist or from expert raters at either a global level, considering whole sessions, or a specific level, considering specific events or segments of particular sessions. The two most common methods used are: (a) therapist and patient rating the session as a whole (Barret-Lennard, 1962; Orlinsky & Howard, 1966; Truax & Mitchell, 1971; Stiles, 1980), and (b) expert raters rating audio or video tapes of sessions with a more limited focus (Goodman & Dooley, 1976; Hill, 1978; Shapiro *et al*, 1984). A more recent development combines the advantages of both approaches (Elliot, 1979; Elliot *et al*, 1982; Barkham & Shapiro, 1986). This utilises the technique of Interpersonal Process Recall (IPR) developed by Kagan (Kagan, 1980; Baiker, 1985). This method involves playing back the session to the therapist and/or patient who then records, often by rating on a scale of helpfulness (Elliot, 1984), their feelings about specific events during the session. These events are then coded using standard rating scales by trained observers.

Global measures

The Barret-Lennard Relationship Inventory (RI; Barret-Lennard, 1962) is among the most widely used questionnaires in process research (Gurman, 1977). It is based on Rogerian theory and rates 85 items on a six-point scale covering level of regard, empathic understanding, congruence, unconditionality and willingness to be known. Each of these can be scored as subscales; the empathy scale is probably the most widely used. The revised version of the RI contains 64 items covering four variables – 'willingness to be known' is no longer included as it lacked predictive power in relation to therapeutic outcome (Gurman, 1977). Internal and test–retest reliability is high. The scale is designed to be rated by either the therapist or patient and separate forms are available.

Truax & Carkhuff (1967) developed observer-rated scales to measure accurate empathy, unconditional positive regard and therapist genuineness. The Accurate Empathy Scale is a nine-point anchored scale evaluating the extent to which the therapist is sensitive to the current feelings and thoughts of the patient, has the ability to communicate his/her awareness of these and has the ability to communicate on the patient's level. Non-possessive warmth rates on a five-point scale the therapist's ability to be non-judgemental and caring. Genuineness rates also on a five-point scale the extent to which the therapist is sincere and non-defensive. There is a large body of work using these scales, relating the three dimensions to outcome, but more recently the psychometric properties and construct validity of these scales have been questioned (Chinsky & Rappaport, 1970; Mitchell *et al*, 1977). It would appear that the relationship between accurate empathy, non-possessive warmth, genuineness and psychotherapy outcome is not as clear cut as was once thought (Gomes-Schwartz, 1978; Lambert *et al*, 1978).

The Therapy Session Report (TSR; Orlinsky & Howard, 1966) was developed to study the experiences of the patient and therapist during the course of a session. This is a structured response questionnaire administered to either patient or therapist after the end of a session. The therapist's form has 152 items and takes 10 to 15 minutes to complete. The ten areas covered include six focusing on the patient's experience (self-adaption, behaviour, feelings, concerns, motives and dialogue) and four on the therapist's experience (aims, behaviour, feelings, session development and evaluation). The TSR has been factor analysed on many dimensions (Orlinsky & Howard, 1977) including facet factors, session factors, sequence factors and person factors. They constructed a typology of global-session experience based on the factors of patient distress and therapist effectiveness and proposed four session types, using sailing metaphors to describe them: smooth sailing, heavy going, foundering, and coasting.

Stiles (1980) has also studied the impact of individual psychotherapy sessions (as distinct from measuring outcome after a long series of sessions). He developed the Session Evaluation Questionnaire (SEQ) which is completed by both patient and therapist after individual sessions. This consists of 22 bipolar adjective scales presented in a seven-point semantic differential format. The first 11 adjective pairs concern the feelings about the session, for example safe–dangerous, slow–fast, and the last 11 pairs the feelings after the session, for example happy–sad, confident–angry. The SEQ is quick to rate (two minutes) and to score (one minute) and is therefore more applicable than the TSR for repeated measures. Stiles describes two distinct dimensions, depth/value and smoothness/ease with moderately high therapist/patient agreement. His suggested typology shows a great deal of agreement with that of Orlinsky & Howard (1977). He describes four types of sessions (continuing the sailing metaphor) as shallow and rough, shallow and smooth, deep and rough, and deep and smooth.

The Vanderbilt Psychotherapy Process Scale (VPPS; Gomes-Schwartz, 1978) was developed from the TSR for use by external raters who score entire sessions or selected segments lasting 10–15 minutes. The measures are seen as a compromise between global impressions of a full session and focused impressions of a single behaviour or communication. The original VPPS developed by Strupp (Gomes-Schwartz & Schwartz, 1978), consisting of 84 items rated on a Likert-type scale, has been factor analysed (Gomes-Schwartz, 1978) to give seven internally consistent scales, rating therapist and patient behaviour and attitudes. These are: patient exploration, therapist exploration, patient participation, patient hostility, therapist warmth and friendliness, negative therapist attitude and therapist directiveness. The VPPS has been used to study the impact of different therapeutic styles (Gomes-Schwartz, 1978; Gomes-Schwartz & Schwartz, 1978) on outcome and is a psychometrically sound instrument. Inter-rater reliability is fairly good for both patient ($r = 0.79$) and therapist items ($r = 0.75$).

The Vanderbilt Negative Indicators Scale (VNIS; Strupp *et al*, 1981) was designed for independent observers to rate patient and therapist activity thought to be predictive of poor outcome in brief psychotherapy. It is a 42-item scale grouped into five sections: patient personal qualities and attitudes, therapist personal qualities and attitudes, errors in technique, patient–therapist interaction and a global scale. Each is rated on a six-point scale. Preliminary data indicate satisfactory levels of inter-rater reliability and the ability to distinguish between good and poor outcome (Sachs, 1983).

The Therapeutic Alliance Scale (Marziali *et al*, 1981) rates both positive and negative factors in patients and therapist. It concentrates on the affective, attitudinal aspects rather than specific responses, techniques or actions. This is a 42-item scale, 21 items referring to therapist, 21 to patient attitudes, with examples of positive and negative attitudes. Each item has an operational definition and is rated on an 'intensity of presence' scale from 0 to 5 by trained observers. Two subscales, therapist total contribution scale and patient total contribution scale, were obtained and have high internal consistency. Inter-rater reliability is good for both patient ($r = 0.76$) and therapist items ($r = 0.82$). Patient contribution scores distinguish between poor and good outcome, and patient and therapist self-report forms have been developed (Marziali, 1984).

The Therapist Action Scale (TAS) and Patient Action Scale (PAS) (Hoyt *et al*, 1981) focus directly on what patients and therapists actually do within psychotherapy sessions and are based on previous work on activity within therapy sessions (Malan, 1963; Goodman & Dooley, 1976; Horowitz, 1979; Hoyt, 1979). The 24 (PAS) and 25 (TAS) items are rated as having occurred or not, and if an item has occurred, a rating of emphasis in relation to the overall activity within the session is made on a five-point scale by expert observers. In general both inter-rater and test–retest reliability were good ($r = 0.75$–0.87 for both scales), although there was poor agreement on whether the activity occurred or not and this suggests a need for more precise definition of threshold. These scales have not yet been widely used in outcome studies, but as they are easy to use and assess specific discrete items they deserve further study.

The Patient Experiencing Scale (Klein *et al*, 1969) and the Therapist Experiencing Scale (Klein & Mathieu-Coughlan, 1984) have been used for global and specific ratings of process. They are based on the work of Rogers (1959) and Gedlin (1962), and are designed for trained raters observing segments of therapy sessions. According to Klein *et al* (1969), 'experiencing' refers to the ''quality of an individual's experiencing of himself, the extent to which his ongoing, bodily, felt flow of experiencing is the basic datum of his awareness and communications about himself, and the extent to which this inner datum is integral to action and thought''.

The Patient Experiencing Scale has seven anchored points of experiencing, rated on content and treatment. The points range from 1, where the patient talks only of external events with no mention of self, through 4, where feelings and experiences are discussed, to 7, where experiencing is easily presented. The Therapist Experiencing Scale, also on a seven-point scale, records the 'referent' and 'manner' dimensions. The referent dimension concerns the aspect of the client's experiencing that is influenced by the therapist's words, and the manner dimension judges the therapist's level of experiencing – how experientially involved he is in the dialogue. Most work with these scales has used the patient's form (Klein & Mathieu-Coughlan, 1984). It has a manual with standardised training techniques (Klein *et al*, 1969) and has been used with either clinically naive or sophisticated judges. Once trained, inter-rater reliability is good.

Specific process measures

There have been many studies looking at specific events in psychotherapy ranging from patient variables to therapist variables. Many rating scales have been developed, often for a particular study, and rate events (e.g. number of silences, number of interpretations) with little attention paid to the psychometric properties of the instruments. In recent years there has been an increased interest in 'verbal response modes' using well developed methods of rating, and examples of these are presented here. More extensive reviews of specific process scales are given by Greenberg & Pinsoff (1986).

Response modes are a category of language behaviour that imply a particular interpersonal intent (Stiles, 1978) and are distinguished from content categories, which code the semantic meaning of verbal utterances, and extralinguistic categories, which code specific speech features (Russel & Stiles, 1979) such as pitch and rate (e.g. the Client Vocal Quality Scale; Rice & Koke, 1981).

Response-mode analysis is usually based on a common set of five major variables: question, 'advisement' (consideration/deliberation), reflection, interpretation and self-disclosure. Goodman & Dooley (1976) reviewed the necessary criteria for the categorisation of these modes and use the above categories plus silence. Similar systems have been developed by Hill (1978), Stiles (1978), Elliot (1979) and Shapiro *et al* (1984). Shapiro *et al*'s (1984) Modified Behaviour Rating System is based on the Elliot Helper Behaviour Rating System, as this is considered to define its categories in terms that are closer to clinical concepts of therapist behaviour than the other systems. Their modified system has 12 categories: closed question, open question, process advisement, general advisement, reflection, interpretation, reassurance, disagreement, self-disclosure, information, exploration, and other. 'Exploration' is seen as incorporating a category intermediate between interpretation and reflection, and captures the shared frame of reference characterised by negotiation implied by the conversational model of psychotherapy (Hobson, 1985).

In order for verbal response modes to be rated by trained observers, sessions are divided into 'response units', usually grammatical sentences, which are then classified into modes of response. Satisfactory levels of inter-rater reliability have been reported. Verbal response modes have been widely used to distinguish between therapists of different schools (Stiles, 1979; Hardy & Shapiro, 1985) and to study the relationship with empathy using interpersonal process recall (Barkham & Shapiro, 1986). Because they do not depend on a particular theoretical orientation, they offer an excellent way of comparing what psychotherapists of different persuasions actually do, and they highlight factors particularly relevant to outcome.

References

AMERICAN PSYCHIATRIC ASSOCIATION (1980) *Diagnostic and Statistical Manual of Mental Disorders* (3rd edn). Washington, DC: APA.

ANASTASI, A. (1968) *Psychological Testing*. Toronto: Macmillan.

AUERBACH, A. H. (1983) Assessment of psychotherapy outcome from the viewpoint of expert observer. In *The Assessment of Psychotherapy Outcome* (eds M. Lambert, E. R. Christensen & S. S. DeJulio). New York: Wiley-Interscience.

——, LUBORSKY, L. & JOHNSON, M. (1972) Clinicians' prediction of psychotherapy outcome: a trial of a prognostic index. *American Journal of Psychiatry*, **128**, 830–835.

BAIKER, C. P. (1985) Interpersonal process recall in clinical training and research. In *New Developments in Clinical Psychology* (ed. F.N.Watts), pp. 262–283. Chichester: Wiley.

BARKHAM, M. & SHAPIRO, D. A. (1986) Counselor verbal response modes and experienced empathy. *Journal of Consulting Psychology*, **33**, 3–10.

BARRET-LENNARD, G. T. (1962) Dimensions of therapist response as causal factors in therapeutic change. *Psychological Monographs*, **76**, 562.

BARRON, F. (1953) An ego-strength scale which predicts response to psychotherapy. *Journal of Consulting Psychology*, **17**, 327–333.

BATTLE, C. C., IMBER, S. D., HOEHN-SARIC, R., *et al* (1966) Target complaints as criteria of improvement. *American Journal of Psychotherapy*, **20**, 184–192.

BEUTLER, L. E. & CRAGO, M. (1983) Self-report measures of psychotherapy outcome. In *The Assessment of Psychotherapy Outcome* (eds M. Lambert, E. R. Christensen & S. S. DeJulio). New York: Wiley-Interscience.

BOND, G., BLOCH, S. & YALOM, I. D. (1979) The evaluation of a "target problem" approach to outcome measurement. *Psychotherapy: Theory, Research and Practice*, **16**, 48–54.

BONI, G., BLOCH, S. & YALOM, I. D. (1979) The evaluation of a 'target problem' approach to outcome measurement. *Psychotherapy: Theory, Research and Practice*, **16**, 48–53.

BUTLER, J. & HAIG, G. (1954) Changes in the relation between self-concepts and ideal concepts consequent upon client centered counseling. In *Psychotherapy and Personality Change* (eds C. R. Rogers & R. Dymond), pp. 55–75. Chicago: University of Chicago Press.

CALSYN, R. J. & DAVIDSON, W. S. (1978) Do we really want a program evaluation strategy based on individual goals? A critique of goal attainment scaling. *Evaluation Studies: Review Annual*, **1**, 700–713.

CHINSKY, J. M. & RAPPAPORT, J. (1970) Brief critique of the meaning and reliability of 'accurate empathy' ratings. *Psychological Bulletin*, **73**, 379–380.

CROOK, T., HOGARTY, G. E. & ULRICH, R. F. (1980) Inter-rater reliability of informants' ratings. Katz Adjustment Scales R Form. *Psychological Reports*, **47**, 427–432.

DAHLSTROM, W. G., WELSH, G. S. & DAHLSTROM, L. E. (1972) *An MMPI Handbook, vol. 1. Clinical Applications* (revised edn). Minneapolis: University of Minnesota Press.

DAVIDSON, C. V. & DAVIDSON, R. H. (1983) The significant other as data source and data problem in psychotherapy outcome research. In *The Assessment of Psychotherapy Outcome* (eds M. Lambert, E. R. Christensen & S. S. DeJulio). New York: Wiley-Interscience.

DEROGATIS, L. R. (1976) *Scoring and Procedures. Manual for PAIS*. Baltimore: Clinical Psychometric Research.

—, LIPMAN, R. S., RICKELS, K., *et al* (1974) The Hopkins Symptom Checklist (HSCL). A measure of primary symptom dimensions. In *Psychological Measurements in Psychopharmacology: Modern Problems in Pharmacopsychiatry*, vol. 7. (ed. P. Pichot), pp. 79–110. Basel: Karger.

DEWITT, K. N., KALTREIDER, N. B., WEISS, D. S., *et al* (1983) Judging change in psychotherapy. Reliability of clinical formulations. *Archives of General Psychiatry*, **40**, 1121–1128.

ELLIOT, R. (1979) How clients perceive helper behaviours. *Journal of Consulting Psychology*, **26**, 285–294.

— (1984) A discovery-orientated approach to significant change events in psychotherapy: interpersonal process recall and comprehensive process analysis. In *Patterns of Change. Intensive Analysis of Psychotherapy Process* (eds L. N. Rice & L. S. Greenberg). New York, Guilford Press.

—, BARKER, C. B., CASKEY, N., *et al* (1982) Differential helpfulness of counselor verbal response modes. *Journal of Consulting Psychology*, **29**, 354–361.

ELLSWORTH, R. B. (1975) Consumer feedback in measuring the effectiveness of mental health programs. In *Handbook of Evaluation Research*, vol. 2 (eds M. Guttentag & E. L. Struening), pp. 239–274. Beverly Hills, California: Sage Publications.

ENDICOTT, J., SPITZER, R. L., FLEISS, J. L., *et al* (1976) The Global Assessment Scale. A procedure for measuring overall severity of psychiatric disturbance. *Archives of General Psychiatry*, **33**, 766–771.

— & — (1978) A diagnostic interview – the Schedule for Affective Disorders and Schizophrenia. *Archives of General Psychiatry*, **35**, 837–844.

EXNER, J. E. (1978) *The Rorschach. A Comprehensive System, vol. 2. Current Research and Advanced Interpretation*. New York: Wiley.

EYSENCK, H. G. & EYSENCK, S. B. G. (1969) *Personality Structure and Measurement*. San Diego: R. R. Knapp.

FISKE, D. W. (1975) The use of significant others in assessing the outcome of psychotherapy. In *Psychotherapy Change Measures* (eds I. E. Waskow & M. B. Parloff), DHEW, no. 74-120. Washington, DC: US Government Printing Office.

GARFIELD, S. L. (1978) Research on client variables in psychotherapy. In *Handbook of Psychotherapy and Behaviour Change. An Empirical Analysis* (eds S. L. Garfield & A. E. Bergin). New York, Wiley.

GEDLIN, E. T. (1962) *Experiencing and the Creation of Meaning*. New York: Free Press of Glencoe.

GLAZER, W. M., AARONSON, H. S., PRUSOFF, B. A., *et al* (1980) Assessment of social adjustment in chronic ambulatory schizophrenics. *Journal of Nervous and Mental Diseases*, **168**, 493–497.

GLESER, G. C. (1975) Evaluation by psychological tests. In *Psychotherapy Change Measures* (eds I. E. Waskow & M. B. Parloff), DHEW, no. 74-120. Washington, DC: US Government Printing Office.

GOMES-SCHWARTZ, B. (1978) Effective ingredients in psychotherapy. Prediction of outcome from process variables. *Journal of Consulting and Clinical Psychology*, **46**, 1023–1035.

— & SCHWARTZ, J. M. (1978) Psychotherapy process variables distinguishing the 'inherently helpful' person from the professional psychotherapist. *Journal of Consulting and Clinical Psychology*, **46**, 196–197.

GOODMAN, G. & DOOLEY, D. (1976) A framework for help-intended interpersonal communication. *Psychotherapy: Theory, Research and Practice*, **13**, 106–117.

GORDON, C. (1969) Self conception methodologies. *Journal of Nervous and Mental Diseases*, **148**, 328–364.

GREEN, B. L., GLESER, G. L., STONE, W. N., *et al* (1975) Relationships among diverse measures of psychotherapy outcome. *Journal of Consulting and Clinical Psychology*, **43**, 689–699.

GREENBERG, L. & PINSOFF, W. (eds) (1986) *The Psychotherapeutic Process*. New York: Guilford.

GURLAND, B. J., YORKSTON, N. J., STONE, A. R., *et al* (1972) The Structured and Scaled Interview to Assess Maladjustment (SSIAM). A description, rationale and development. *Archives of General Psychiatry*, **27**, 259–264.

GURMAN, A. S. (1977) The patient's perception of the therapeutic relationship. In *Effective Psychotherapy. A Handbook of Research* (eds A. S. Gurman & A. M. Razin). Oxford: Pergamon Press.

—— & RAZIN, A. M. (eds) (1977) *Effective Psychotherapy. A Handbook of Research*. Oxford: Pergamon Press.

GYNTHER, M. D. & GREEN, S. B. (1982) Methodological problems in self-report. In *Handbook of Research Methods in Clinical Psychology* (eds P. C. Kendall & J. N. Butcher), pp. 355–428. New York: Wiley.

HARDY, G. E. & SHAPIRO D. (1985) Therapist response modes in prescriptive versus exploratory psychotherapy. *British Journal of Clinical Psychology*, **24**, 235–245.

HATHAWAY, S. R. & McKINLEY, J. C. (1967) *Minnesota Multiphasic Personality Inventory: Manual for Administration and Scoring*. New York: Psychological Corporation.

HERSEN, M. & BELLACK, A. (1976) *Behavioural Assessment: A Practical Handbook*. New York, Pergamon.

HILL C. E. (1978) Development of a counselor verbal response category system. *Journal of Consulting Psychology*, **25**, 461–468.

HOBSON, R. F. (1985) *Forms of Feeling: The Heart of Psychotherapy*. London: Tavistock Press.

HOROWITZ, M. J. (1979) *States of Mind*. New York: Plenum.

——, WILNER, N. & ALVAREZ, W. (1979) Impact of event scale: a measure of subjective stress. *Psychosomatic Medicine*, **41**, 209–218.

——, WEISS, D. S., KALTREIDER, N., *et al* (1984) Reactions to the death of a parent: results from patients and field subjects. *Journal of Nervous and Mental Disease*, **172**, 383–392.

——, MARMAR, C. R., WEISS, D. S., *et al* (1986) Comprehensive analysis of change after brief dynamic psychotherapy. *American Journal of Psychiatry*, **143**, 582–589.

HOYT, M. F. (1979) Aspects of termination in a time-limited brief psychotherapy. *Psychiatry*, **42**, 208–219.

——, MARMAR, C. R., HOROWITZ, M. J., *et al* (1981) The Therapist Action Scale and the Patient Action Scale. Instruments for the assessment of activities during dynamic psychotherapy. *Psychotherapy: Theory, Research and Practice*, **78**, 109–115.

KAGAN, N. (1980) Influencing human interaction. Eighteen years with IPR. In *Psychotherapy Supervision: Theory, Research and Practice* (ed. A. K. Hess), pp. 262–283. Chichester: Wiley.

KALTREIDER, N., DeWITT, K., LIEBERMAN, R., *et al* (1981*a*) Individual approaches to outcome assessment: a strategy for psychotherapy research. *Journal of Psychiatric Treatment and Evaluation*, **3**, 105–111.

——, DeWITT, K. N., WEISS, D. S., *et al* (1981*b*) Patterns of individual change scales. *Archives of General Psychiatry*, **38**, 1263–1269.

KAPPES, B. M. & PARISH, T. S. (1979) The personal attribute inventory: a measure of self-concepts and personality profiles. *Educational and Psychological Measurement*, **39**, 955–958.

KATZ, M. M. & LYERLY, S. B. (1963) Methods for measuring adjustment and social behaviour in the community: 1 Rationale, description, discriminative validity and scale development. *Psychological Reports*, **13** (monograph suppl. 4–V13), 503–555.

KIRESUK, T. J. & SHERMAN, R. E. (1978) Goal attainment scaling. In *Evaluation of Human Service Programs* (eds C. C. Attkisson, W. A. Hargreaves, M. J. Horowitz & J. Sorenson), pp. 341–371. New York: Academic Press.

KLEIN, M. M., MATHIEU, P. L., GENDLIN, E. T., *et al* (1969) *The Experiencing Scale: A Research and Training Manual*. Madison: University of Wisconsin Extension Bureau of Audiovisual Instruction.

—— & MATHIEU-COUGHLAN, P. (1984) The patient and therapist experiencing scales. In *The Psychotherapeutic Process: A Research Handbook* (eds L. Greenberg & W. Pinsoff). New York: Guilford.

KLOPFER, W. G. (1968) Current status of the Rorschach Test. In *Advances in Psychological Assessment*, vol. 1. (ed. P. McReynolds), pp. 131–149. Palo Alto: California, Science and Behaviour Books.

LAMBERT, M. J. (1983) Introduction to assessment of psychotherapy outcome: historical perspective and current issue. In *The Assessment of Psychotherapy Outcome* (eds M. Lambert, E. R. Christensen & S. S. DeJulio). New York: Wiley-Interscience.

——, DEJULIO, S. S. & STEIN, D. M. (1978) Therapist interpersonal skills: process, outcome, methodological considerations and recommendations for future research. *Psychological Bulletin*, **85**, 467–489.

——, CHRISTENSEN, E. R. & DEJULIO, S. S. (eds) (1983) *The Assessment of Psychotherapy Outcome*. New York: Wiley-Interscience.

——, SHAPIRO, D. A. & BERGIN, A. E. (1986) The effectiveness of psychotherapy. In *Handbook of Psychotherapy and Behaviour Change* (3rd edn) (eds S. L. Garfield & A. E. Bergin). New York: Wiley.

LIPMAN, R. S., COVI, L. & SHAPIRO, A. K. (1979) The Hopkins Symptom Checklist (HSCL). Factors derived from the HSCL–90. *Journal of Affective Disorders*, **1**, 9–24.

LORR, M. (1975) Therapist measures of outcome. In *Psychotherapy Change Measures* (eds I. E. Waskow & M. B. Parloff), DHEW, no. 74–120. Washington, DC: US Government Printing Office.

——, MCNAIR, D. M., MICHAUX, W. W., *et al* (1962) Frequency of treatment and change in psychotherapy. *Journal of Abnormal and Social Psychology*, **64**, 281–292.

—— & MCNAIR, D. M. (1965) Expansion of the interpersonal behaviour circle. *Journal of Personal and Social Psychology*, **2**, 823–830.

LUBORSKY, L. (1962) Clinicians' judgements of mental health. A proposed scale. *Archives of General Psychiatry*, **7**, 407–417.

MALAN, D. H. (1963) *A study of Brief Psychotherapy*. London: Tavistock.

MARZIALI, E. (1984) Three viewpoints on the therapeutic alliance: similarities, differences and association with psychotherapy outcome. *Journal of Nervous and Mental Diseases*, **7**, 417–423.

——, MARMAR, C. & KRUPNICK, J. (1981) Therapeutic Alliance Scales: development and relationship to psychotherapy outcome. *American Journal of Psychiatry*, **138**, 361–364.

MINTZ, J. (1977) The role of the therapist in assessing psychotherapy outcome. In *Effective Psychotherapy. A Handbook of Research* (eds A. S. Gurman & A. M. Razin). Oxford: Pergamon Press.

—— (1981) Measuring outcome in psychodynamic psychotherapy. *Archives of General Psychiatry*, **38**, 503–506.

——, AUERBACH, A. H., LUBORSKY, L., *et al* (1973) Patient's, therapist's and observer's views of psychotherapy. A 'Rashomon' experience or a reasonable consensus? *British Journal of Medical Psychology*, **46**, 83–89.

MITCHELL, K., BOZARTH, J. & KRAUFT, C. (1977) A reappraisal of the therapeutic effectiveness of accurate empathy, non possessive warmth and genuiness. In *Effective Psychotherapy. A Handbook of Research* (eds A. Gurman & A. Razin), pp. 482–502. Oxford: Pergamon Press.

MURRAY, H. A. (1943) *Thematic Apperception Test*. Cambridge, Massachusetts: Harvard University Press.

NEWMAN, E. L. (1983) Therapist's evaluation of psychotherapy. In *The Assessment of Psychotherapy Outcome* (eds M. Lambert, E. R. Christensen & S. S. DeJulio). New York: Wiley-Interscience.

O'MALLEY, P. M. & BACHMAN, J. G. (1979) Self esteem and education. Sex and cohort comparisons among high school seniors. *Journal of Personality and Social Psychology*, **37**, 1153–1159.

ORLINSKY, D. E. & HOWARD, K. I. (1966) *Therapy Session Report, Form T*. Chigago: Institute for Juvenile Research.

—— & —— (1977) The therapist's experience of psychotherapy. In *Effective Psychotherapy: A Handbook of Research* (eds A. S. Gurman & A. M. Razin). Oxford: Pergamon Press.

OVERALL, J. E. & GORHAM, D. R. (1962) Brief Psychiatric Rating Scale. *Psychological Reports*, **10**, 799–812.

PLATT, S. (1981) Social adjustment as a criterion of treatment success: just what are we measuring? *Psychiatry*, **44**, 95–110.

——, WEYMAN, A. J., HIRSCH, S. R., *et al* (1980) The Social Behaviour Assessment Schedule (SBAS): rationale, contents, scoring and reliability of a new interview schedule. *Social Psychiatry*, **15**, 43–55.

REMINGTON, M. & TYRER, P. (1979) The Social Functioning Schedule – a brief semi-structured interview. *Social Psychiatry*, **14**, 151–157.

RICE, L. N. & KOKE, C. J. (1981) Vocal style and the process of psychotherapy. In *Speech Evaluation in Psychiatry* (ed. J. K. Derby). New York: Grune and Stratton.
—— & GREENBERG, L. S. (eds) (1984) *Patterns of Change. Intensive Analysis of Psychotherapy Process.* New York: Guilford Press.
ROGERS, C. R. (1959) A theory of therapy, personality and interpersonal relationships as developed by the client-centred framework. In *Psychology: A Study of a Science: Formulation of the Person and the Social Context*, vol. 3 (ed. S. Koch). New York: McGraw-Hill.
ROSENBAUM, M. (1980) A schedule of assessing self-control behaviors: preliminary findings. *Behavior Therapy*, **11**, 109–121.
ROSENBAUM, R. L. & HOROWITZ, M. J. (1983) Motivation for psychotherapy. A factorial and conceptual analysis. *Psychotherapy: Theory, Research and Practice*, **20**, 346–354.
ROSENBERG, M. (1965) *Society and the Adolescent Self Image.* Princeton: Princeton University Press.
RUSSEL, R. L. & STILES, W. B. (1979) Categories for classifying language in psychotherapy. *Psychological Bulletin*, **86**, 404–419.
SHAPIRO, D. A., BARKHAM, M. & IRVING, D. L. (1984) The reliability of a modified helper behaviour rating system. *British Journal of Medical Psychology*, **57**, 45–48.
SACHS, J. S. (1983) Negative factors in brief psychotherapy: an empirical assessment. *Journal of Consulting and Clinical Psychology*, **51**, 557–564.
SHOSTROM, E. L. (1966) *Manual: Personal Orientation Inventory.* San Diego: Educational and Industrial Testing Service.
SLOANE, R. B., STAPLES, F. R., CRISTOL, A. H., *et al* (1975) *Psychotherapy Versus Behavior Therapy.* Cambridge, Massachusetts: Harvard University Press.
SPITZER, R. L., ENDICOTT, J., FLEISS, J. L., *et al* (1970) The Psychiatric Status Schedule. A technique for evaluating psychopathology and impairment in role functioning. *Archives of General Psychiatry*, **23**, 41–55.
——, WILLIAMS, J. B. W. & GIBBON, M. (1985) *Instruction Manual for the Structured Clinical Interview for DSM–III–R (SCID).* New York: Biometrics Research Department, New York State Psychiatric Institute.
STILES, W. B. (1978) Verbal response modes and dimensions of interpersonal roles: a method of discourse analysis. *Journal of Personality and Social Psychology*, **36**, 693–703.
—— (1979) Verbal response modes and psychotherapeutic technique. *Psychiatry*, **42**, 49–62.
—— (1980) Measurement of the impact of psychotherapy sessions. *Journal of Consulting and Clinical Psychology*, **48**, 176–185.
STORROW, H. A. (1960) The measurement of outcome in psychotherapy. *Archives of General Psychiatry*, **2**, 142–146.
STRUPP, H. H. & BLOXOM, A. L. (1975) Therapist's assessment of outcome. In *Psychotherapy Change Measures* (eds I. E. Waskow & M. B. Parloff), DHEW, No. 74–120. Washington, DC: US Government Printing Office.
—— & HADLEY, S. W. (1977) A tripartite model of mental health and therapeutic outcomes with special reference to negative effects in psychotherapy. *American Psychologist*, **32**, 187–196.
—— & —— (1979) Specific vs non-specific factors in psychotherapy – a controlled study of outcome. *Archives of General Psychiatry*, **36**, 1125–1136.
——, MORAS, K., SANDELL, J., *et al* (1981) Vanderbilt negative indicators scale: an instrument for the indentification of deterrents to progress in time limited dynamic psychotherapy. Unpublished manuscript, Vanderbilt University, Nashville.
TRAMONTANA, M. G. & SHERRETS, S. D. (1983) Assessing outcome in disorders of childhood and adolescence. In *The Assessment of Psychotherapy Outcome* (eds M. J. Lambert, E. R. Christensen & S. S. DeJulio). New York: Wiley-Interscience.
TRUAX, C. B. & CARKHUFF, R. R. (1967) *Toward Effective Counselling and Psychotherapy.* Chicago: Aldine Publishing.
—— & MITCHELL, K. M. (1971) Research on certain therapist interpersonal skills in relation to process and outcome. In *Handbook of Psychotherapy and Behaviour Change* (eds A. E. Bergin & S. L. Garfield). New York: Wiley.
WASKOW, I. E. & PARLOFF, M. B. (1975) *Psychotherapy Change Measures*, DHEW, no. 74–120. Washington, DC: US Government Printing Office.
WEISS, D. S., HOROWITZ, M. J. & WILNER, N. (1974) The Stress Response Rating Scale: a clinician's measure for rating the response to serious life events. *British Journal of Clinical Psychology*, **23**, 202–215.

——, DeWitt, K. N., Kaltreider, N. B., *et al* (1985) A proposed method for measuring change beyond symptoms. *Archives of General Psychiatry*, **42**, 703–708.

Weissman, M. M. (1975) The assessment of social adjustment. A review of techniques. *Archives of General Psychiatry*, **32**, 357–365.

—— & Paykel, E. S. (1974) *The Depressed Woman: A Study of Social Relationships*. Chicago: University of Chicago Press.

—— & Bothwell, S. (1976) The assessment of social adjustment by patient self report. *Archives of General Psychiatry*, **33**, 1111–1115.

——, Sholomskas, D. & John, K. (1981) The assessment of social adjustment. An update. *Archives of General Psychiatry*, **38**, 1250–1258.

Wing, J. K., Cooper, J. E. & Sartorius, N. (1974) *Measurement and Classification of Psychiatric Symptoms*. Cambridge: Cambridge University Press.

Zilberg, N. J., Weiss, D. S. & Horowitz, M. J. (1982) Impact of Event Scale: a cross-validation study and some empirical evidence supporting a conceptual model of stress response syndromes. *Journal of Consulting and Clinical Psychology*, **50**, 407–414.

11 Rating scales for special purposes. II: Child psychiatry and eating disorders

SIOBHAN MURPHY and PETER TYRER

In recent years there has been a proliferation in rating scales for use in child and adolescent psychiatry. The use of semistructured interviewing techniques was pioneered by Rutter & Graham (1968) and has been refined in line with DSM–III (American Psychiatric Association, 1980) diagnostic criteria more recently. This chapter is primarily concerned with instruments that are usually appropriate only with children or adolescents. For reasons of space only a selected review is possible and this is confined to those ratings that are likely to be carried out primarily by psychiatrists. Information about the assessment of intelligence and many aspects of child performance are not discussed and are to be found in standard texts on child psychology.

Some of the common questions asked by trainee psychiatrists involved in child psychiatric research are presented in Table 11.1. Before deciding that this chapter is appropriate for a particular need, the research worker should establish whether the problem under scrutiny is one that is truly specific to child psychiatry. If not, there are likely to be other scales mentioned in previous chapters that could be equally; if not more, appropriate for the investigation.

Developmental and family data

There are a number of checklists which have been used for the collection of demographic data. Many have been developed with a particular interest in mind and there does not appear to be a single instrument which has been used by a number of investigators.

The Early Clinical Drug Evaluation Unit (ECDEU) Paediatric Packet developed a comprehensive questionnaire, the Children's Personal Data Inventory (Guy, 1976). This did not contain details of family psychiatric history or pre- and perinatal data. Cambell (1977) has developed a template which includes family psychiatric and medical history, pre- and perinatal and early-life data. While these used together are comprehensive, they lack validity or reliability studies.

TABLE 11.1
Guide to use of rating instruments in child psychiatry

Primary need	Relevant instruments
To examine factors predisposing to childhood psychiatric disorder	See under 'Developmental and family data'
To establish diagnostic status	See under 'Diagnostic rating scales'
Studies of autistic children	See under 'Assessment of interaction and communication' and 'Behavioural assessment'
Assessment of social function	See under 'Behavioural assessment'
To monitor progress in general therapy	See under 'Behavioural assessment' and 'Emotional disorders'
To study progress in psychotherapy and and family therapy	See under 'Assessment of interaction and communication' and see rating instruments in psychotherapy (p. 176)
To record anxiety, depression, obsessional symptoms and eating problems	See under 'Emotional disorders' and 'Eating disorders'

The Research Obstetrical Scale (ROS) is a 27-item checklist containing six pre-natal, 13 delivery and eight neonatal events (Sameroff *et al*, 1982). Subscores of each category and a total (summed) score are obtained. This has been used in prospective studies and has differentiated children diagnosed with infantile autism from those diagnosed with schizophrenia (Green *et al*, 1984). It does not contain the variable 'maternal bleeding', which is included in the Rieder *et al* (1977) scale for pre- and perinatal factors.

An alternative method for collecting family data is the family history (Endicott *et al*, 1975). In this method, established rating scales are used to obtain psychiatric histories of families. Psychiatric illness has been noticed to be under-reported using Research Diagnostic Criteria (Feighner *et al*, 1972), but accuracy is increased if more informants are used (Andreasen *et al*, 1977). The Developmental Profile (Alpern *et al*, 1980) was designed to assess differences in the pattern and level of development in children from birth to nine years. It can be administered by lay personnel to parents who give yes/no answers to a series of developmentally sequenced items that tap skills and abilities on five scales: physical, self-help, social, academic, and communication. A developmental age is obtained from each scale in six-monthly intervals to three and half years and yearly intervals after.

Assessment of interaction and communication

Family communication has been assessed using the Parent–Adolescent Communication Inventory (Bienvenu, 1969) and the Marital Communication Inventory (Bienvenu, 1970) by Ro-Trock *et al* (1977) in a study comparing individual and family therapy. The Parent–Adolescent Communication

TABLE 11.2
Diagnostic schedules

Name	Reference	Main points
Children's Assessment Schedule (CAS)	Hodges & McKnew (1982)	Semistructured; manual; 128 items; for ages 7–16 years; 45–60 min; clinician rater/assessed; current or last 6 months; not for schizophrenia or Axis II
Diagnostic Interview for Children and Adolescents (DICA)	Herjanic & Reich (1982)	Structured; 267–311 items; for ages 6–17 years; 60–90 min; computer scored; lay interview or clinician; current episode assessed; not for schizophrenia or Axis II
Diagnostic Interview Schedule for Children (DISC)	Costello *et al* (1984)	Highly structured; 264–302 items; for ages 6–17 years; 50–70 min; lay interviewer/ clinician; computer scored; past year assessed; rates schizophrenia, not Axis II
Interview Schedule for Children (ISC)	Kovacs (1980–81)	Semistructured; over 200 items; for ages 8–17 years; 60–90 min; clinician rater; assessments at 2 weeks or 6 months; rates schizophrenia and Axis II
Kiddie–SADS (K–SADS)	Puig-Antich *et al* (1978)	Semistructured; over 200 items; for ages 6–17 years; 45–120 min; clinician rater; rates schizophrenia, not Axis II

Inventory is designed to be a self-report form for adolescents. It has 36 items scored on a three-point scale of frequency of occurrence and has satisfactory psychometric data. The Marital Communication Inventory is a 48-item self-report measuring the patterns, characteristics and styles of marital communication. It is scored on a four-point scale of frequency of occurrence, and has high reliability.

Diagnostic rating scales

Rutter & Graham's scale (1968) was the first to use the child as an informant in making a diagnosis. This was developed for 7–12-year-olds with norms available for 10–12-year-olds. In a semistructured interview information is collected on 24 items including five on motor abilities and attention, six on relationships and 12 on observed and reported affect. An overall rating of psychiatric state (normal, mild, definite) and a diagnosis are made, based on clinical judgement. Reliability and validity data are satisfactory although the inter-rater agreement is higher for the presence of psychiatric illness than for the individual diagnoses.

Following Rutter and Graham's example a number of semistructured diagnostic screening instruments have been developed (Orvaschel, 1985).

The following have been developed for different populations and, therefore, have different emphases. All of them have been widely tested and developed and provide DSM–III Axis I diagnoses. They use both parent and child as informants and have extensive psychometric information available (Table 11.2).

The Children's Assessment Schedule (CAS; Hodges *et al*, 1982) is a semistructured interview designed initially to study psychosomatic illness. It can be used as a clinical or research tool with children aged 7–16; children and parents are interviewed separately. The first part is a 75-item semistructured interview based on a wide range of feelings and behaviour occurring in the last six months. The second part rates onset and duration of positive symptoms using information from the first part, and the third part consists of 53 observation items. It can be scored as a total problem score, a symptom-specific score or a symptom-complex score. Scoring and additional information are contained in the available manual. Psychometric data are satisfactory. The major problem with using the CAS is that no method of resolving disagreement between parent and child informants is given.

The Diagnostic Interview for Children and Adolescents (DICA; Herjanic & Reich, 1982) is a highly structured schedule. It can be used with children aged 6–17 and has a separate parental form. The first part is a joint interview with parents and child covering 19 areas of baseline and demographic information. The second part is conducted separately, and consists of 247 questions which are grouped around clinical disorders allowing separate diagnoses to be made. There are eight observational categories in the children's interview and parental interviews include information on pregnancy, infancy, medical history and siblings. Diagnosis is separately derived by computer from parent and child responses and no method of combining information from both is provided. Parent–child agreement on less concrete items has been rather low but is reported to have been improved (Orvaschel, 1975).

The Diagnostic Interview Schedule for Children (DISC; Costello *et al*, 1984, unpublished) was designed for large-scale epidemiological surveys and can be used by trained lay interviewers (Orvaschel, 1975). It is a very highly structured schedule designed for children between 6 and 17 with a separate parents' form (DISC–P). A manual is available and DSM–III Axis I diagnoses are derived by computer. The child questionnaire contains 264 items covering behaviour and symptoms over the last year and is rated on a four-point scale of occurrence. The 302-item parental questionnaire contains further questions on elective mutism, stereotyped movement disorders, pervasive developmental disorders and dissociative disorders. Inter-rater reliability is high; test–retest and parent–child agreement is variable depending on age and type of disorder. Agreement between DISC and DISC–P diagnosis and clinical assessments is poor.

The Interview Schedule for Children (ISC; Kovacs, 1980–81) was developed to assess childhood depression and comprises a core interview and addenda which together give DSM–III Axis I and many Axis II diagnoses. A follow-up ISC is available to assess change. An initial unstructured interview is followed by 43 questions on depressive symptoms. Presence and severity of symptoms are rated on an eight-point anchored scale. The core interview of 100 questions also covers psychotic symptoms and developmental milestones. Most symptoms are rated for the previous two weeks. Acting out is rated for the last six months. Diagnoses are based on a combination of information from parent and child ratings and are formed by clinical consensus. Inter-rater reliability is good, and variation in child–parent agreement in general is a function of observable versus internal symptoms.

The Kiddie SADS (K–SADS; Chambers *et al*, 1985) was developed as a children's version of the Schedule for Affective Disorders and Schizophrenia (SADS; Endicott & Spitzer, 1978 – see Chapter 9) for studies in childhood depression. It is a semistructured questionnaire for children between 6 and 17 which must be administered by a trained clinician. Parents and child are interviewed separately. The initial relatively unstructured part records information on onset and duration. Part 2 includes questions on approximately 200 specific symptoms and behaviours. Part 3 includes observational items and a global assessment (Schaffer *et al*, 1985). Items are rated on a six- to seven-point anchored scale for severity in both the last week and during the worst period of the present episode. Responses are recorded for each informant and final ratings made by clinicians integrating these ratings with clinical judgement.

Past history can be judged using K–SADS–E (epidemiological version) (Orvaschel *et al*, 1982). This includes Axis I disorders plus attention deficit, substance abuse and suicidal behaviour. K–SADS has satisfactory inter-rater reliability and is sensitive to change (Puig-Antich *et al*, 1978). Test–retest reliability is fair for depression, good for conduct disorders and poor for psychotic symptoms and anxiety states.

These diagnostic scales all have individual strengths and weaknesses. The choice between them will depend on the investigator's particular interests, needs and resources.

Behavioural assessment

Most of the rating scales developed to measure change in observable behaviour have been designed for use in drug studies. On the whole they measure only aberrant behaviour and it is thus not possible to tell whether response to treatment by a reduction in inappropriate behaviour is associated with any change in more appropriate behaviour, for example peer relationships.

These scales have been comprehensively reviewed (Conners, 1985; Orvaschel & Walsh, 1984) and only a selection is described here, to illustrate aspects of their use (Table 11.3).

TABLE 11.3
Behaviour checklists

Name	Reference	Main points
Conners Parent Rating Scale	Conners (1970)	Main version has 93 items; for ages 6–14 years; 10–15 min; parent rater; norms for ages 6–14; computer scoring possible; conduct, emotional disorders, school adjustment rated
Conners Parent Rating Scale Revised version	Goyette *et al* (1978)	48 items; for ages 3–17 years; 5–10 min; parent rater; norms for ages 3–17; content as above but not phobias or obsessive/compulsive ratings
Conners Teachers Questionnaire	Conners (1969)	39 items; age range not reported; teacher rater; 5–10 min; norms for ages 4–12; rates conduct, anxiety and school development
Conners Teachers Questionnaire Revised Revised	Goyette *et al* (1978)	28 items; for ages 3–17 years; teacher rater; 5–10 min; norms for ages 3–17; rates conduct disorders
Child Behaviour Checklist	Achenbach & Edelbrock (1983)	138 items; for ages 3–16 years; parent rater; 15–20 min; norms for ages 3–16; rates conduct, emotional disorders (not phobias) and social adjustment
ADD–H Comprehensive Teacher Rating Scale (ACTeRS)	Ullman *et al* (1984)	24 items; for ages 5–12 years; teacher rater; 5–10 min; norms for ages 5–12; rates hyperactivity, attention, oppositional and social adjustment behaviours
Werry–Weiss–Peters Activity Rating Scale (WWP)	Werry (1968)	31/32 items; age range not reported; parent rater; 5–10 min; norms for ages 2–9; rates hyperactivity
Personality Inventory for Children	Wirt (1977)	240/131 items; for ages 3–16 years; parent rater; 20–45 min; norms for ages 3–16; rates conduct, emotional, psychotic behaviour, cognitive development, social and school adjustment and family problems; does not rate somatic complaints, phobias, obsessive–compulsive disorders

The Conners Parent Rating Scale is available in the original form (Conners, 1970) and in a shortened form (Goyette *et al*, 1978). The original is a 93-item checklist, grouped into 24 general categories completed by parents, of behaviour in the last month, scored on a four-point scale from 'not at all' to 'very much'. The weighted items are summed to give a total symptom score. The following stable factors have emerged from factor analysis: conduct problem, anxiety, impulsive/hyperactive, learning problem, psychosomatic, perfectionism, antisocial attitudes, and muscle tension. The shortened form has 48 items and has norms for ages 3–17. There is no assessment of depression or severe disorders (e.g. psychoses, Gilles de la Tourette syndrome). Because these scales show a practice effect between the first and second administration (Werry & Sprague, 1974), more than two baseline administrations are recommended (Conners & Barkley, 1985).

The Conners Teacher Questionnaire (TQ; Conners, 1969) is a 39-item symptom list completed by the class teacher on a four-point scale as above.

This covers three broad areas: classroom behaviour, group participation and attitude towards authority. Factor analysis yields four factors: conduct problem, inattentive/passive, tension/anxiety and hyperactivity. This is also available in a shortened version of 28 items (Goyette *et al*, 1978). A ten-item abbreviated version of the Teacher Questionnaire can be used when repeated measures are needed from parents or teachers (Goyette *et al*, 1978).

The Child Behaviour Checklist (Achenbach & Edelbrock, 1983) is a 138-item parent-rated scale. The scales were derived from factor analysis of checklist responses by parents of children referred to mental health services. Extensive normative data are available. Factor scores can be derived for at least eight or nine behaviour scales depending on the age of the child. There is also a social competence scale. Test–retest, inter-rater and internal-consistency reliability data are available. There is also a teacher's version and self-report version for children over 11.

The ADD–H: Comprehensive Teacher Rating Scale (ACTeRS; Ullman *et al*, 1984) was designed to study attention deficit disorder (ADD). This has 24 items rated on a five-point scale from 'almost never' to 'almost always'. The scale covers four areas: inattention, overactivity, social competence, and oppositional behaviour. There are separate scales and norms for boys and girls. This scale has been used to diagnose and monitor treatment in ADD, has high internal consistency and inter-rater reliability.

The Werry–Weiss–Peters Checklist (WWP) has also been used to monitor children's activity in a variety of home settings (Werry, 1968). It records parents' ratings of levels of activity on 32 items. Psychometric data available are very varied and it is recommended that this should be used in addition to other scales and not as a single measure.

The Personality Inventory for Children (Wirt *et al*, 1977) is a general-purpose instrument developed for personality assessment, with subscales covering a wide range of emotional and behavioural problems. It consists of three validity scales, one screening scale and 12 clinical scales. It has many similarities with the Minnesota Multiphasic Personality Inventory (MMPI) although it is rated by an observer, not self-rated. The individual scales provide an assessment of general adjustment and informant response style, cognitive development and academic performance, family cohesion and personality and include: somatic concern, depression, delinquency, withdrawal, anxiety, psychosis, hyperactivity and social skills. Psychometric data are satisfactory (Lachar & Gdowski, 1979).

The Jessness Inventory (Jessness, 1972; Graham, 1981) is a self-report measure of personality and psychopathology. It is a 155-item scale with 11 empirically derived scales including: social maladjustment, value orientation, immaturity, autism, alienation, manifest aggression, withdrawal/depression, social anxiety, repression, denial, and an asocial index. The asocial index has been used as a predictor of delinquency (Jessness, 1972) although its sensitivity with neophyte offenders is variable (Shark & Handal, 1977; Graham, 1981).

TABLE 11.4
Emotional disorders

Name	Reference	Main points
Children's Manifest Anxiety Scale–Revised	Reynolds & Richmond (1978)	Self-report; 28 anxiety items; 9 lie items; for ages 7–16 years; 10–20 min
Bellevue Index of Depression (BID)	Petti (1978)	Semistructured interview; 40 subjective items; for ages 6–16 years; 15–20 min
Children's Depression Rating Scale and revised version (CDRS, CDRS–R)	Poznanski (1979, 1984)	Semistructured interview; 17 items, including 3 observed items; for ages 6–12 years; 30 min
Children's Depression Inventory (CDI)	Kovacs (1981)	Self-report; 27-item scale; measure of severity; for ages 6–17
Reynolds Adolescent Depression Scale (RADS)	Reynolds (1985)	Self-report; 30-item scale; extensive norms; for ages 12–18 years; 10 min
Leyton Obsessional Inventory Child version	Berg *et al* (1986)	Card-sort task; 44-item scale; for ages 8–18; measures of resistance and interference

Emotional disorders

The appropriate scales are summarised in Table 11.4, but see also Table 11.2.

Anxiety

The diagnosis and treatment of anxiety in children has not been researched as extensively as in adults and scales for measuring anxiety suffer from a number of methodological flaws. Many of the scales have been developed for adults and are used in either modified or unchanged forms, so their validity is uncertain for children. It is clear that fears and anxieties are common in children but most measures do not distinguish between symptomatic and non-symptomatic levels of anxiety or do not include norms. The most extensively researched scales are the subscales of the diagnostic interviews. The CAS rates all the Axis I anxiety disorders, DICA rates all except generalised anxiety and panic, DISC and ISC rate all except generalised anxiety, and K–SADS all except avoidance.

The Children's Manifest Anxiety Scale (Reynolds & Richman, 1978), a self-report scale, has been revised to a scale of 'what I think, what I feel'. This measures 37 statements of anxiety symptoms and lie statements and has established norms for school-age children. It is scored either yes or no. Reliability data are acceptable. The lie scales reflect age and are highest with young children. The test takes 20–45 minutes to complete.

Depression

Childhood depression has been more extensively studied, and there are a number of reviews of available instruments (Reynolds, 1984; Petti, 1985;

Strober & Werry, 1986) and diagnostic criteria (Poznanski *et al*, 1985). All the diagnostic interviews (see above) have subscales for rating depression; the ISC was developed specifically for use in childhood depression. K-SADS-P (present episode) has been used as a screening device and as an instrument to measure change (Puig-Antich *et al*, 1983).

The Bellevue Index of Depression (Petti, 1978) is a semistructured interview administered separately to both the parents and child. It has 40 items falling into ten categories rated on a scale of 0–3 based on severity of problem. It is easily scored, short to administer (15–20 minutes) and has high reliability. It does however depend on self-report and cannot be easily transposed to DSM–III diagnosis.

The Children's Depression Rating Scale (CDRS; Poznanski *et al*, 1979) and its revised version (CDRS–R; Poznanski *et al*, 1984) are being widely used, often in combination with the self-report measure, the Children's Depression Inventory (CDI; Kovacs, 1980–81) (see below). The CDRS and CDRS–R can be used with children aged 6–12 in a semistructured clinical interview. The 17-item scale contains 14 items rated on verbal responses and three items rated on observed behaviour, for example depressed affect, tempo of language and hypoactivity. Scales are scored from 1 to 7 and 1 to 5 for sleep, appetite and tempo of speech. This rating system runs from normal (1) to degrees of abnormality (5–7). It has been used as a screening device with a cut-off score for major depression. It does not allow other DSM–III criteria to be transposed, but it is easy and quick to administer and has good reliability.

There are also a number of self-report scales available; the CDI (Kovacs, 1980–81; Saylor *et al*, 1984) is probably the most widely used. All self-report ratings, depending as they do on a child's ability to describe depressive feelings, may have high numbers of false negative responses (Petti & Law, 1982). The CDI was initially developed from the Beck Depression Inventory (BDI) for adults (Beck, 1967) and identifies moderate to severe depression with good reliability. It is not a diagnostic measure, merely a measure of severity. There are quite marked between-group differences in score and it should not be used as a screening device on its own. However, within psychiatric out-patient groups it does distinguish between diagnosis reached using the ISC covering the last two weeks (Kovacs, 1985). It is a 27-item symptom-orientated scale. Each item is rated from 0 to 2 and a total summed score is obtained.

The P–CDI (Garber, 1984) is a parental form of the CDI with the first 27 items being identical. Parents are asked to rate how they feel their child feels. An additional eight items asks how the parents feel about their child. It correlates with the CDI, is internally consistent and has an acceptable test–retest reliability.

The self-report Reynolds Adolescent Depression Scale (RADS; Reynolds, 1984) correlates well with other measures (e.g. the BDI), and has good reliability and internal consistency. It is easy and quick to administer (ten minutes), consisting of 30 statements which are scored on a four-point scale of frequency of occurrence. It also inquires directly about mood in the last week.

The Leyton Obsessional Inventory–Child Version (Berg *et al*, 1986) was developed from the Leyton Obsessional Inventory for Adults (Cooper, 1970) as a card-sort task. It has been shown to be sensitive to change (Flament *et al*, 1985) and has demonstrated reliability (Berg *et al*, 1986). It consists of 44 symptom cards which are sorted into 'yes' and 'no' responses. The total number of 'yes' responses produces the symptom score. 'Yes' response cards are then scored on a weighted five-point scale of resistance and a four-point scale of interference. This scale is suitable for ages 8 to 18.

Eating disorders

Rating scales in anorexia nervosa and bulimia nervosa have flourished recently as the syndrome has become more widely reported. Many investigators have developed their own eating-disorder questionnaires with little psychometric investigation. The following are some of the most commonly used scales plus a new rating scale for bulimia with acceptable psychometric properties.

The majority of the frequently used scales are self-report scales. The major problem with these is the anorectic's pervasive denial of illness (Halmi, 1985). They therefore have limitations as screening or diagnostic procedures but may be used to assess change. The most widely used is the Eating Attitudes Test (EAT; Garner & Garfinkel, 1979). This is a 40-item test – the items are specifically concerned with feelings and behaviour in anorexia, not bulimia. It has been used as a screening tool to identify clinical and subclinical cases of anorexia (Garner & Garfinkel, 1979; Button & Whitehouse, 1981) but has very variable positive predictive value (Halmi, 1985).

The Eating Disorder Inventory (EDI; Garner *et al*, 1983) is a more comprehensive measure of eating disorders and covers a wider range of attitudes and behaviour, including bulimia. It is a 64-item scale with eight subscales: drive for thinness, bulimia, maturity fears, body dissatisfaction, ineffectiveness, perfectionism, interpersonal distress and interoceptive awareness. Each scale is scored separately. It was validated on a population of anorectics and did not include DSM–III criteria of binge eaters.

The Binge Scale Questionnaire (Hawkins & Clement, 1980) was designed to provide both descriptive and quantifiable information about behaviour and attitudes in binge eating. It is a 19-item questionnaire, with nine items used to calculate the score. It can measure severity but is not a diagnostic scale.

The Binge Eating Questionnaire (Halmi *et al*, 1981) includes both all the items on the DSM–III criteria for bulimia and Russell's (1970) criteria for bulimia nervosa. A diagnosis of bulimia is made by a positive answer to all of the criteria questions for bulimia.

The Bulimic Investigatory Test, Edinburgh (BITE; Henderson & Freeman, 1987) was designed to identify binge eaters in epidemiological surveys and to provide clinical information on cognitive and behavioural aspects of the disorder. It includes DSM–III and Russell's (1970) descriptions of bulimia. It is a 33-item self-report with two subscales, a symptom scale and a severity scale. It has good reliability and high internal consistency.

The Slade Anorexic Behavioural Scale (Slade, 1973) is an observer scale designed for in-patients. It is a 22-item scale of characteristic anorectic behaviours which are marked as present or absent. It has high inter-rater reliability and can differentiate between patient and control groups. It is not used as a diagnostic scale but as a rating of behaviour occurring in a given situation. The total score is the sum of 'yes' responses.

References

ACHENBACH, T. M. & EDELBROCK, C. S. (1983) *Manual for the Child Behaviour Checklist and Revised Child Behaviour Profile*. Burlington, V. E.: Thomas M. Achenbach.

ALPERN, G. D., BOLL, T. J. & SHEARER, M. S. (1980) *Developmental Profile II: Manual*. Aspen Colo: Psychological Development Publications.

AMERICAN PSYCHIATRIC ASSOCIATION (1980) *Diagnostic and Statistical Manual for Mental Disorders* (3rd edn) (DSM–III). Washington, DC: APA.

ANDREASEN, N. C., ENDICOTT, J., SPITZER, R. L., *et al* (1977) The family history method using diagnostic criteria. *Archives of General Psychiatry*, **34**, 1229–1235.

BECK, A. T. (1967) *Depression: Clinical Experimental and Theoretical Aspects*. New York: Harper and Row.

BERG, C. J., RAPOPORT, J. L. & FLAMENT, M. (1986) The Leyton Obsessional Inventory–Child Version. *American Academy of Child Psychiatry*, **25**, 84–91.

BIENVENU, M. J. (1969) Measurement of parent–adolescent communication. *Family Co-ordinator*, **18**, 117–121.

—— (1970) Measurement of marital communication. *Family Co-ordinator*, **1**, 26–31.

BUTTON, E. J. & WHITEHOUSE, A. (1981) Subclinical anorexia nervosa. *Psychological Medicine*, **11**, 509–516.

CAMBELL, M. (1977) Demographic parameters of disturbed children: a template to the CPDI and CSU. Its rationale and significance. *Psychopharmacology Bulletin*, **13**, 30–33.

CHAMBERS, W., PUIG-ANTICH, J., HIRSCH, M., *et al* (1985) The assessment of affective disorder in children and adolescents by semistructured interview: test–retest reliability of the K–SADS–P. *Archives of General Psychiatry*, **42**, 696–702.

CONNERS, C. K. (1969) A teacher rating scale for use in drug studies with children. *American Journal of Psychiatry*, **126**, 884–888.

—— (1970) Symptom patterns in hyperkinetic neurotic and normal children. *Child Development*, **41**, 667–682.

—— (1985) Methodological and assessment issues in pediatric psychopharmacology. In *Psychopharmacology in Childhood and Adolescence* (2nd edn) (ed. J. M. Weiner). New York: John Wiley & Son.

—— & BARKLEY, R. A. (1985) Rating scales and checklists for child psychopharmacology. *Psychopharmacology Bulletin*, **21**, 809–851.

COOPER, J. (1970) The Leyton Obsessional Inventory. *Psychological Medicine*, **1**, 48–64.

ENDICOTT, J., ANDREASEN, N. & SPITZER, R. L. (1975) *Family History–Research Diagnostic Criteria*. New York: Biometrics Research, New York State Psychiatric Institute.

—— & SPITZER, R. L. (1978) A diagnostic interview: the SADS. *Archives of General Psychiatry*, **35**, 837–853.

FEIGHNER, J. P., ROBINS, E., GUZE, S. B., *et al* (1972) Diagnostic criteria for use in psychiatric research. *Archives of General Psychiatry*, **26**, 57–63.

FLAMENT, M. F., RAPAPORT, J. L., BERG, C. J., *et al* (1985) Clomipramine treatment in childhood obsessive–compulsive disorder: a double-blind controlled study. *Archives of General Psychiatry*, **42**, 977–983.

GARBER, J. (1984) The developmental progression of depression in female children. In *Childhood Depression, New Directions for Child Development* (eds D. Achetti & K. Schneider-Rosen), pp. 29–58. San Francisco: Jossey Bass.

GARNER, D. M. & GARFINKEL, P. E. (1979) The eating attitudes test: an index of the symptoms of anorexia nervosa. *Psychological Medicine*, **9**, 273–279.

——, OLMSTEAD, M. P. & POLLUY, J. (1983) Development and validation of a multi-dimensional eating disorder inventory for anorexia nervosa and bulimia. *International Journal of Eating Disorders*, **2**, 15–34.

GOYETTE, C. H., CONNERS, C. K. & ULRICH, R. F. (1978) Normative data on Revised Conners Parent and Teachers Rating Scales. *Journal of Abnormal Child Psychology*, **6**, 221–236.

GRAHAM, S. A. (1981) Predictive and concurrent validity of the Jessness Inventory Asocial Index: when does a delinquent become a delinquent? *Journal of Consulting and Clinical Psychology*, **49**, 740–742.

GREEN, W. H., CAMBELL, M., HARDESTY, A. S., *et al* (1984) A comparison of schizophrenic and autistic children. *Journal of the American Academy of Child Psychiatry*, **23**, 399–409.

GUY, W. (1976) *ECDEV Assessment Manual for Psychopharmacology (revised)*. Publication no. (ADM) 76–338. Rockville, Maryland: Department of Health, Education and Human Welfare.

HALMI, K. (1985) Rating scales in the eating disorders. *Psychopharmacology Bulletin*, **21**, 1001–1003.

——, FALK, J. R. & SCHWARZ, E. (1981) Binge eating and vomiting: a survey of a college population. *Psychological Medicine*, **11**, 697–706.

HATHAWAY, S. R. & McKINLEY, J. C. (1967) *The Minnesota Multiphasic Personality Inventory: Manual for Administration and Scoring*. New York: Psychological Corporation.

HAWKINS, R. C. & CLEMENT, P. F. (1980) Development and construct validation of a self-report of binge-eating tendencies. *Addictive Behavior*, **5**, 219–226.

HENDERSON, M. & FREEMAN, C. P. L. (1987) A self-rating scale for bulimia, the 'BITE'. *British Journal of Psychiatry*, **100**, 18–24.

HERJANIC, B. & REICH, W. (1982) Development of a structured psychiatric interview for children: agreement between child and parent on individual symptoms. *Journal of Abnormal Child Psychology*, **10**, 307–324.

HODGES, K., McKNEW, D., CYTRYN, L., *et al* (1982) The Child Assessment Schedule (CAS) diagnostic interview: a report on reliability and validity. *Journal of the American Academy of Child Psychiatry*, **21**, 468–473.

JESSNESS, C. F. (1972) *The Jessness Inventory (Revised)*. Palo Alto, California: Consulting Psychologists Press.

KOVACS, M. (1980–81) Rating scales to assess depression in school-age children. *Acta Paedopsychiatrica*, **46**, 305–315.

—— (1985) The Children's Depression Inventory. *Psychopharmacology Bulletin*, **21**, 995–998.

LACHAR, D. & GDOWSKI, C. L. (1979) *Actuarial Assessment of Child and Adolescent Personality. An Interpretive Guide for the Personality Inventory for Children Profile*. Los Angeles: Western Psychological Services.

ORVASCHEL, H. (1985) Psychiatric interviews suitable for research with children and adolescents. *Psychopharmacology Bulletin*, **21**, 737–802.

——, PUIG-ANTICH, J., CHAMBERS, W., *et al* (1982) Retrospective assessment of child psychopathology with the Kiddie–SADS–E. *Journal of the American Academy of Child Psychiatry*, **21**, 392–397.

—— & WALSH, G. (1984) *The Assessment of Adaptive Functioning in Children: A Review of Existing Measures Suitable for Epidemiological and Clinical Services Research*. Monograph for NIMH series, no. 3, DHHS Publication no. (ADM), 84–1343. Washington, DC: US Government Printing Office.

PETTI, T. A. (1978) Depression in hospitalized child psychiatry patients: approaches to measuring depression. *Journal of the American Academy of Child Psychiatry*, **17**, 49–59.

—— (1985) Scales of potential use in the psychopharmacologic treatment of depressed children and adolescents. *Psychopharmacology Bulletin*, **21**, 951–955.

—— & LAW, W. (1982) Imipramine treatment of depressed children: a double-blind study. *Journal of Clinical Psychopharmacology*, **2**, 107–110.

POZNANSKI, E. O., COOK, S. C. & CARROLL, B. J. (1979) A depression rating scale for children. *Pediatrics*, **64**, 442–450.

——, GROSSMAN, J. A., BUCHSBAUM, Y., et al (1984) Preliminary studies of the reliability and validity of the Children's Depression Rating Scale. *Journal of the American Academy of Child Psychiatry*, **23**, 191–197.

——, MOKROS, H. D., GROSSMAN, J., et al (1985) Diagnostic criteria in childhood depression. *American Journal of Psychiatry*, **142**, 1168–1173.

PUIG-ANTICH, J., BLAU, S., MARX, N., et al (1978) Prepubertal major depressive disorders: a pilot study. *Journal of the American Academy of Psychiatry*, **17**, 695–707.

——, CHAMBERS, W. J. & TAMBRIZI, M. A. (1983) The clinical assessment of current depressive episodes in children and adolescents: interviews with parents and children. In *Affective Disorders in Childhood and Adolescence: An Update* (eds D. P. Cantwell & G. A. Carlson), pp. 157–179. New York: SP Medical and Scientific Books.

REYNOLDS, C. R. & RICHMAN, B. D. (1978) What I think and feel: a revised measure of children's manifest anxiety. *Journal of Abnormal Child Psychology*, **6**, 271–280.

REYNOLDS, W. M. (1984) Depression in childhood and adolescents: phenomenology, evaluation and treatment. *School Psychological Reviews*, **13**, 171–182.

RIEDER, R. O., BROMAN, S. U. & ROSENTHAL, D. (1977) The offspring of schizophrenics. *Archives of General Psychiatry*, **34**, 789–799.

RO-TROCK, G. K., WELLISCH, D. & SCHOOLAR, J. (1977) A family therapy outcome study in an inpatient setting. *American Journal of Orthopsychiatry*, **47**, 514–522.

RUSSELL, G. (1979) Bulimia nervosa: an ominous variant of anorexia nervosa. *Psychological Medicine*, **9**, 429–448.

RUTTER, M. & GRAHAM, P. (1968) The reliability and validity of the psychiatric assessment of the child. I. Interview with the child. *British Journal of Psychiatry*, **114**, 563–579.

SAMEROFF, A. J., SELFER, R. & ZAX, M. (1982) Early development of children at risk for emotional disorder. *Monographs of the Society for Research in Child Development*, **47** (7, serial no. 199), 1–82.

SAYLOR, C. F., FINCH, A. J., Jr, SPIRITO, A., et al (1984) The Children's Depression Inventory: a systematic evaluation of psychometric properties. *Journal of Consulting and Clinical Psychology*, **52**, 955–967.

SCHAFFER, O., GOULD, M. S., BRASIC, J., et al (1985) A Children's Global Assessment Scale (CGAS) (for children 4 to 16 years of age). *Psychopharmacology Bulletin*, **21**, 747–748.

SHARK, M. L. & HANDAL, P. J. (1977) Reliability and validity of the Jessness Inventory: a caution. *Journal of Consulting and Clinical Psychology*, **45**, 692–695.

SLADE, P. D. (1973) A short anorexic behaviour scale. *British Journal of Psychiatry*, **122**, 83–85.

STROBER, N. & WERRY, J. S. (1986) The assessment of depression in children and adolescents. In *Assessment of Depression* (eds N. Sartorius & T. A. Ban). Heidelberg: Springer-Verlag.

ULLMAN, R. K., SLEATOR, E. K. & SPRAGUE, R. L. (1984) A new rating scale for diagnosis and monitoring of ADD children (ACTeRS). *Psychopharmacology Bulletin*, **29**, 160–164.

WERRY, J. S. (1968) Developmental hyperactivity. *Pediatric Clinics of North America*, **15**, 581–599.

—— & SPRAGUE, R. L. (1974) Methylphenidate in children–effect of dosage. *Australian and New Zealand Journal of Psychiatry*, **8**, 9–19.

WIRT, R. B., LACHAR, D., KLINEDINST, J. K., et al (1977) *Multidimensional Description of Child Personality: A Manual for the Personality Inventory for Children*. Los Angeles: Western Psychological Services.

12 Writing up research

PETER TYRER and CHRIS FREEMAN

The maxim 'publish or perish' used to hang like the sword of Damocles over every ambitious young doctor. The phrase is unfortunate because it implies that all publications are of value, no matter how tawdry or uninformative they happen to be. Nevertheless, it is obvious that good research work has to be published if it is ever to be perceived as good research. This is not an easy process. Some trainees entertain the fond hope that a well executed research project with clear conclusions will somehow write itself. Of course the evidence lies in the data and no amount of clever writing can raise the status of a shoddy study, but it is still extremely easy to write a bad paper even when the study procedure is excellent.

Trainees often ask the question, 'When shall I start writing up my project?' If they have carried out the project correctly they will have already started writing it up, because a good protocol gives the main reasons for carrying out the research and the methods to be employed. This protocol can be used as a basis to develop the subsequent paper to be submitted to a journal showing the main findings of the study. Before the first data are collected it is a useful exercise to record your expectations of the final results. It is an unfortunate fact that research workers tend to find what they expect to find. This does not mean that they are necessarily biased, but when the results are very different from those that are expected it is worthy of special note. As the study progresses it should be noted whether there are any deviations from the original protocol and whether the predictions in the original documents have been shown to be correct. There are bound to be variations and these can be written into the embryonic paper before any data are analysed.

Sometimes the deviations from the protocol are so great that the study has to be abandoned. Even this may not be a disaster. Research psychiatrists are nothing if not enterprising and it may be felt that the abandonment of the project has important lessons for us all and so publication is achieved (e.g. Blackwell & Shepherd, 1967; Cook *et al*, 1988). However, most studies do not turn out to be disastrous and they progress steadily, sometimes exceedingly slowly, towards their goal. A critical time follows the analysis of the data. Investigators almost always like to see positive results, partly because most studies set out to disprove null hypotheses, but also because investigators (rightly) perceive that positive results are easier to publish than negative ones. Nevertheless, one should not be too disappointed if the results are negative; it is sometimes said that a universal set of negative results is much more valuable than the more common finding of a few islands of positive results that are only just visible in a sea of uniform negative findings. The tendency is then to overstate the positive findings and come to incorrect conclusions. Once the findings have been analysed fully, three questions need to be asked. Is the study worth publishing? If so, who would be most interested in the findings? How many papers are going to be needed?

Is the study worth publishing?

The answer to this question should usually be a positive one and should not normally be dependent on the results of the study. One of the criticisms of scientific investigators is that they tend to find the results they want to find and if the results are at variance with this expectation they are in some way considered as wrong. Unexpected results are usually of much more interest than expected ones and the trainee should not be inhibited from making appropriate conclusions and reporting them to the profession. There could be other reasons why the study is not worth publishing but almost all of these should have been appreciated long before the results were analysed. If the study deviated fundamentally from the original protocol it may be beyond recovery, but the analysis of the findings should not affect the decision as to whether or not it is published. If the numbers are too small (a common error with trainees with limited time and budgets) no differences are likely to be detected even when they may, in fact, be present. The reasons for this are discussed by Dr Johnson in Chapter 2.

It is sometimes difficult to decide whether a study is worth publishing if it merely replicates the findings of earlier studies. This in itself is not a reason for not publishing, because a number of studies carried out in different settings that come to the same conclusions successively add weight to the findings. However, if the study concerns a subject that has already been extensively investigated and methodologically it is less satisfactory than previous work, then it is unlikely to add much to the literature. Again, however, this question should have been asked early in the study, before data were collected.

Who would be most interested in the findings?

This important question is sometimes forgotten. It is natural that research workers would like the whole world to read about their findings after they have invested so much time and effort into creating them, but the sad fact is that only a small minority of papers have genuine general interest and most are looking for a small, specialised readership. It is often valuable to take advice from a more experienced investigator before selecting which journal to send the paper to. This is likely to avoid disappointment that will follow from sending a paper first to a general journal and then to progressively more specialised journals with diminishing circulations in the hope that one will eventually accept the work. An experienced editor can detect without much difficulty a paper that has been submitted many times previously. It does not appear to have been specifically for the journal and its format is often not in the appropriate style. This can lead to a paper being rejected which might well have been accepted if it had been written specifically for that journal in the first instance.

How many papers are going to be needed?

The correct answer to this question is 'as few as possible'. There is a tendency for investigators to publish more articles than is necessary. In the long term this is counterproductive as it adds needlessly to the world literature on the topic and the good articles tend to be hidden among the bad. There are many reasons why investigators publish too many articles, including the natural wish to beef up a curriculum vitae with as many publications as possible, suitable acknowledgement to coworkers by giving them 'first-author status' in subsidiary articles, and the wish to spread the information among as wide a readership as possible by publishing in different places. None of these can be defended; numbers of publications are no substitute for quality, and the international citation of published articles makes similar or over-lapping articles unnecessary.

There may sometimes be occasions in which several papers are necessary to describe one piece of work. These usually involve large-scale studies that either have such a volume of information that it cannot all be presented in one article, or where there are important differences in the data (e.g. of time-scale, nature or measurement) that justify more than one publication.

Preparation of papers

All journals have their idiosyncrasies and it is important to recognise these when preparing papers. The final version of the paper should be written with a copy of the journal's 'instructions to authors' as its constant companion. Particular attention will need to be paid to the reference format. Although more journals are now using the Vancouver convention for reference format, there are still many minor variations which are often easy to miss. Close examination of previous articles published in the journal will help to illustrate the style and emphasis of contributions likely to be accepted. Brevity is almost always desirable. Bernard Shaw once apologised to a correspondent, "I am sorry this letter is so long, I did not have time to write a shorter one," and the same could apply with even more force to many papers published in the scientific literature.

It is important to confine the article to the subject matter of the inquiry. A research article is not a review of the literature and there is no need for a vast array of references that are of general interest only. The introduction should set the problem in perspective and explain the reasons behind the study, the section on methods should give a clear and concise account of how the study was undertaken in a way that enables easy replication, and the results should be described clearly, with a balance achieved between figures (which have the main visual impact), tables and textual descriptions. It is important when describing results to confine the account to the significant findings and not to point out trends that do not reach significance. Care should also be taken not to duplicate results in figures, tables and text; this adds unnecessary length to the article. Finally, the discussion section of the paper needs to be relevant and should not meander whimsically over the whole territory covered by the research work. If the study was worthwhile, it will have implications and it is these that need to be discussed fully in the discussion section.

There are many books and articles devoted to the writing up of scientific papers (e.g. Crammer, 1978). Two recently published papers are essential reading (*British Medical Journal*, 1988, 1989). The former is a set of guidelines, regularly published by the *British Medical Journal*, for writing manuscripts submitted to biomedical journals. This latest publication has a number of changes and gives a list of all the journals which subscribe to this scheme. The 1989 paper also gives much useful help in this area, and it reproduces the checklists which the *British Medical Journal* sends to assessors, which are an invaluable guide when starting to write a paper.

Submission of the manuscript

Before the final manuscript is submitted to the journal of choice, it is advisable to show it to at least one colleague with more experience in the subject. After many hours of loving care devoted to preparation it is a chastening experience to have a paper dissected after what appears to be inadequate perusal. Nevertheless, initial impressions count a great deal and a badly written paper of excessive length creates a long-lasting negative impression before its contents have been properly evaluated. Particular care needs to be taken with the summary of the findings. Journals often confine the length of these to a set number of words and it is a hard task to compress the main findings into this limit. The summary is probably the most important part of the paper because it is (unfortunately) the only part that

TABLE 12.1
Checklist of points necessary before submitting a manuscript

Feature	Important aspects
Length	Be concise – most good original contributions can be covered in under 3000 words
Relevance	Do not include material that is outside the scope of your inquiry
Summary	Ensure it is comprehensive and of the right length
Format	Follow slavishly the instructions to authors
References	Make sure these are in appropriate journal style
Statistics	Some journals now insist on certain tests being carried out on data (e.g. confidence limits as well as probabilities). Check before submitting the manuscript
Duplication	Avoid repeating information in tables, figures and texts. Also be careful not to repeat the findings of your other published papers; if a manuscript is too similar to another published one it is likely to be rejected
Comprehension	Is the paper understandable? Test this by giving it to someone who has no special knowledge of the subject concerned. It should still be readily understood
Acknowledgements	Some journals limit these severely. Try not to be too wordy or effusive

most people are going to read. A number of papers published in other journals are also based largely on summaries, although in recent years more care has been taken over this and the authors of the paper may sometimes be asked to contribute their own brief résumés of a published article.

A checklist of important points that will need attention before a manuscript is submitted is given in Table 12.1. Many of these will appear to be self-evident but will still need to be addressed. For example, if a non-specialist reads the article and cannot understand it, do not be too ready to dismiss the subject as beyond the reader's capabilities. Might it be that the article has too many Greco-Latin polysyllables, contains too much unnecessary jargon, or has just a touch of patronising pomposity that marks it out as only for the few who are in the know? Copy editors at all medical publishers spend a large part of their time simplifying unnecessarily convoluted material to make it understandable as well as using valuable publication space more economically.

When the manuscript has been through all its checks and revisions it is ready to go to the editor of the chosen journal, together with the required number of photocopies indicated in the instructions for authors. It is often helpful to explain to the editor in your covering letter why you think your paper is suited for the journal. All editors like to feel that there is a particular reason for their journal being selected for submission, and in most cases this will be true. If so, put it into words, and if a little flattery also creeps into the letter it will not do any harm. Remember, the editor has to make the final decision about publication of the manuscript. Although he/she will be guided in large part by the assessors of the paper, if the paper comes into the hinterland between acceptance and rejection, the editor's influence will be considerable. If you have made an excellent case that the material in your paper would be out of place elsewhere, it may well sway the editor in your favour.

There is often an uncomfortably long gap between acceptance of a paper and the date of publication. If this seems to be getting too long, do not be afraid to chivvy the journal staff and ask when the paper will be published. It is not unknown for papers to get lost in editorial offices, and if their authors do not complain, no one else will. When the galley or page proofs arrive, check them carefully for errors but avoid the temptation of making new changes that differ entirely from the original manuscript. Sometimes it may be permitted to add new material as a 'note added at proof' if this is particularly germane, but it will need a persuasive argument to get it accepted.

Psychiatrists over the years have led to several stereotypes in the public mind. One is that of dogmatic wordiness unsubstantiated by facts. The research worker in psychiatry is in an excellent position to quash this unrepresentative impression; good writing will help to eliminate it entirely.

References

BLACKWELL, B. & SHEPHERD, M. (1967) Early evaluation of psychotropic drugs in man: a trial that failed. *Lancet*, *ii*, 819–823.

BRITISH MEDICAL JOURNAL (1988) Uniform requirements for manuscripts submitted to biomedical journals. *British Medical Journal*, **296**, 401–405.

—— (1989) Guidelines for writing up papers. *British Medical Journal*, **298**, 40–42.

COOK, C. H., SCANNELL, T. D. & LIPSEDGE, M. S. (1988) Another trial that failed. *Lancet*, *i*, 524–525.

CRAMMER, J. L. (1978) How to get your paper published. *Bulletin of the Royal College of Psychiatrists*, **2**, 112–113.

13 Using computers in research

CHRIS FREEMAN

Computer enthusiasts and experienced researchers will tell you that computers are easy to use and will save you a great deal of time. This may be true when you are fully familiar with a particular statistics package, but it certainly is not so at the start. You will almost certainly find yourself wondering why you ever bothered to try to use a computer at all, and unless you have large amounts of data you will probably find that on your first attempt, it will take you longer to learn the system, prepare the data in the correct way, and analyse the results than if you had done the whole thing by hand. For large amounts of data, whether they be studies with many subjects or with a great deal of data per case, then computers are the only real answer. If however you have only 30 or 40 cases and 15 to 20 variables per case you may find it much simpler to do things by hand, using a pocket calculator and paper and pencil. Many calculators can do simple descriptive statistics, carry out χ^2 and t-tests and the equivalent non-parametric tests. With small amounts of data the main reasons for using a computer would be either to learn the system for your future use or to carry out certain statistical manipulations that would be difficult or impossible to do without the aid of a computer.

Even if you decide not to use a computer, it is a good idea to collect and code your data as if it were going to be used in this way. Whatever system you use, you will have to convert all your data into numbers and preparing a proper coding sheet, as described below, allows you to do this in a systematic way.

The steps in using a computer

These are outlined in Fig. 13.1. First you will have to prepare your data in a particular way, and this is dealt with more fully below. Each item of information you collect will need to be converted into a number and 'coded'. Wherever possible, you should arrange for the coding to be part

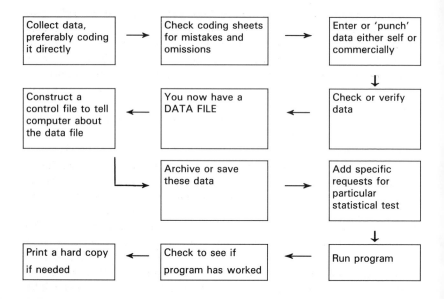

Fig. 13.1   The steps in using a computer to analyse data

of the questionnaire that you are using, rather than have separate coding sheets. Each time you transpose the data, say from your original questionnaire to a coding sheet and then from coding sheet to computer, the chances of errors creeping into the data increase. Even when you are using self-rating questionnaires which are being given to patients, you can arrange for the coding to be down the right hand margin. Once your data have been coded, you will need to check for accuracy to make sure that there are no items of missing data or obvious mistakes, such as people being coded as age 12 when your study protocol declared that the minimum age for entry to the study was 18. Next you have to enter the data on to a computer. If you are using a personal computer (PC), you will have to do this yourself. If you are using a mainframe computer, and especially if you have large amounts of data, it is best to organise this to be done professionally. Entering large amounts of data is very tedious and it really is not cost effective for you to be doing this. There are commercial organisations which will prepare and enter your data, and they will almost certainly do it more accurately than you. For a small extra charge you can ask for your data to be 'verified'. This usually means that the data are entered twice by two separate computer operators and then each item cross-checked by the computer. The term 'punching' is often used for this process. This comes from the time when punch tape or punch cards with small holes in them were used as a means of entering data. The most common computer cards were about seven by three inches and contained 80 columns of data.

Punch cards were put into bundles and read by a mechanical reader into the computer. Although this system is now obsolete, a few punch-card readers are still in use and it is important to be aware of its nature because certain statistical packages still use the 80-column 'card' format even though the cards themselves no longer physically exist (see 'Preparing coding sheets', below).

Once your data have been entered you will have what is called a data file. On a printout this will look just like horizontal columns of figures. The computer can do nothing with these data until it is given instructions about what the figures represent.

You next need to construct a control file. This tells the computer about the data, for example how many cases there are and how many items of information there are for each case, and gives some sort of label to each column so that the computer knows that the figures coded in columns 10 and 11 represent the patient's age, in column 12 the patient's sex, and in column 13 and 14 the patient's psychiatric diagnosis. The ways of constructing this control file vary depending which statistical package you use. In the simplest system, "Minitabs", this system is not used and you give the computer direct instructions each time you want to carry out a statistical manipulation. While this makes things easier in the short term, it does make the system less flexible.

Checking the accuracy of your data

No matter how careful you have been, there will be mistakes in your data. Some mistakes you will never be able to discover. For example, if someone has been coded as age 47 rather than 45, you will not be able to see this mistake, unless you check each item by hand, which will take you as long, if not longer than, entering the data all over again. There are some simple things that you can do. If for example you have left blank columns in your coding of the data, these should form vertical lines on your data file. If there are numbers in these columns then something has been miscoded. A common mistake is for each item of data to be one column out because a key has been pressed twice. You could also make some simple visual checks by hand. For example, if column 43 is where information about in-patient or out-patient status is coded, and you know that in-patients were coded 1 and out-patients coded 2 and no other codes were used, then you can run your eye down that particular column and make sure that it contains only 1s and 2s. Another way of checking your data is to run a program which gives simple descriptive statistics such as maximum and minimum values and range. This will allow you to check that you have no obvious mistakes, such as patients with Hamilton scores of 87 when the maximum score is 40; or patients aged 99 when the oldest subject in your study was 65. Other items are relatively simple to check, for example if your study has 60 subjects, 30 in an experimental group and 30 in control group. Check that the computer has the correct numbers recorded in each group.

Form A   Background Information for Depressive Illness in General Practice Study

Study No.:	0 0 1 7	Cols 1–4
Card No.:	1	Col 5
Interviewer:	3	Col 6

Date of birth (27.2.56) Code as weeks and year   08 5 6   Cols 7–11

Living circumstances
  Lives alone = 1
  Lives with family of origin = 2
  Lives with partner = 3
  Lives with children = 4
  Not known (missing data) = 9   3   Col 12

Educational attainment
  (code number of years of continuous education)
  99 = not known   1 3   Cols 13–14

Who referred for help
  General practitioner = 1
  Other specialist = 2
  Self referral = 3
  Other = 4
  Not known = 9   1   Col 15

Marital status
  Single = 1
  Married = 2
  Separated/divorced = 3
  Widowed = 4
  Not known = 9   2   Col 16

Length of time from GP referral to being seen by
  specialist. Code in number of weeks,

Not applicable,   Code 88
Not known,   Code 99   9 9   Cols 17–18

Number of previous episodes of depression
  None = 1
  1–3 = 2
  4–6 = 3
  More than 7 = 4
  Not known = 9   3   Col 20

Initial Hamilton score
  0–17 items   2 4   Cols 21–22
  18–21 items   0 4   Cols 23–24
  Total score   2 8   Cols 25–28

Fig. 13.2   Example of a coding sheet

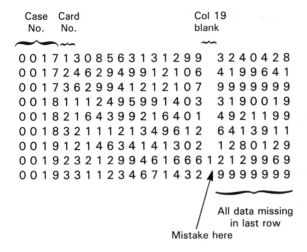

Fig. 13.3   *Example of data file based on coding shown in Fig. 13.2*

Preparing coding sheets

Figure 13.2 gives an example of a coding sheet. It is best to try to collect all your data in this manner and have such sheets prepared at the start of the study, so that data can be entered directly into them. The design illustrated has a number of features.

(a) There are no personal identifiers. In this particular study all personal information, such as name, address, general practitioner, etc., was on a front sheet with clear instructions that that page was to be detached before the data were sent for processing.

(b) All the coding information is down the right-hand margin and all the column boxes lined up beneath each other. This makes the data easier to code and minimises error.

(c) The card number (column 5) refers to the now redundant concept of computer punch cards which used to be the way of feeding information into computers. Although data are now entered directly, many programs still 'think' in terms of cards, each card containing up to 80 columns. You can see from Fig. 13.3 that this study required three cards of data per subject.

(d) It is always best to code the raw information (e.g. date of birth, rather than age). The computer can always work out the age at a later date. In this particular study, we coded only the week and year of birth as we were not interested in the actual day of birth.

(e) It is important to include clear instructions as to how to code various variables on the data sheet (see 'living circumstances', column 12). It is also important to have codes for 'not known' (missing data). If you simply leave a blank you will not be able to determine whether this box was simply not filled in, in error, or whether the information was genuinely not known. It is also important to have categories which are mutually exclusive, for example, in 'living circumstances' it is quite possible for subjects to be living with their family of origin and their partner and with their children, so this item has been badly coded.

(f) For educational attainment, 99 is used for the 'not known' (missing data). This is a two-column variable and it would be impossible for someone to have 99 years of continuous education.

(g) Length of time from GP referral has been coded in number of weeks: it would have been better to have coded the actual dates, in other words date when seen by GP and date when seen by specialist. This gives you much more flexibility in handling your data. It is an unlikely example, but if you wanted to know the patient's age when seen by a GP and age when seen by a specialist, it would be quite difficult to calculate this with the coding as it is laid out in the figure, but relatively easy if you had date of birth, date seen by GP and date seen by specialist.

(h) Column 19 has been left blank. This helps to break up the data into discrete groups and also allows you to check the accuracy of the entering of your data (see Fig. 13.3).

(i) For the number of episodes of depression, the coding sheet has already begun to summarise the data. It would have been much better if the coding had taken two columns and the actual number of previous episodes of depression had been coded. Summarising the data at this early stage loses information. You can always ask the computer to divide the data into subgroups later.

(j) There is unnecessary coding of the initial Hamilton score. It is not strictly necessary to code the total score. You can always ask the computer to add the 0–17 and 18–21 scores together at a later time.

(k) Each page should be clearly numbered, not with a simple page number but with a number that indicates the number of sheets in the coding booklet. It is very easy for a sheet to become detached.

(l) When you are coding data it is best to use a continental seven, with a bar: this will avoid sevens being misread as ones when data are being entered.

Figure 13.3 gives a brief example of what a data file based on the coding sheet in Fig. 13.2 would look like when entered into the computer. This is only a very small part of what would be many rows of figures, each up to 80 columns long. You can see that leaving gaps in the data helps build in some structure and allow you to check for errors.

Using a computer system

Gaining access to a computer is relatively simple with a PC. The software statistical package will be on a floppy disk and will be loaded into the computer each time you use it. If you have a microcomputer with a hard-disk system, then you can store the statistical package on that disk. If you are using a mainframe computer then you will gain access through a terminal. This may be linked directly by a landline to the computer or by a telephone link. PCs themselves can be used as terminals and this is probably the most common installation that you will see.

Computer packages

There are a vast number of statistical and data-handling packages available. Most PCs come with their own statistics package. While some of these are quite adequate, you should be wary of them, as very few were designed specifically for medical/social sciences research. The programmes described below are those most commonly in use; two of them are described in a little more detail because they are the most likely ones that you will come across and the best to use if you are new to using computers to carry out statistical analysis.

The difference between interactive and batch modes

If a program is running in batch mode, it means that, having typed it in on a terminal and asked the computer to run it, the whole program runs at once and you get all your answers back in one 'batch'. If a program is running in interactive mode, then it carries out each command that you type as soon as you have typed it. Usually the signal for it to do this is to press the carriage return on the keyboard. In general, it is much easier to use interactive programs when you are learning. You can recognise your mistakes as you make them and make appropriate corrections.

Minitabs

This is by far the most user-friendly package available, and unless you have large amounts of data to analyse, is the best system to learn first. Minitabs was originally designed in 1972 for students in introductory statistics courses. Since that time it has expanded greatly and will be able to carry out most of the statistical manipulations that you are likely to require. It is available on a wide variety of computers, including micros, minis and mainframes. The system is an interactive one and the commands in Minitabs allow the user to 'speak' to the computer in simple, English-like commands. The commands usually correspond to the main steps that you would follow if you were carrying out the test by hand.

The following is not an exhaustive list of the procedures that Minitabs can carry out, but you may find it useful. It can produce:

(a) displays and summaries of data, such as histograms, dot-plots, scatter plots, etc.

(b) confidence intervals and tests for population means
(c) *t*-tests and analysis of variance
(d) correlation and regression, including multiple regressions
(e) χ^2 tests and contingency tables
(f) a variety of non-parametric statistics, including sign procedures and Wilcoxon signed-rank procedures.

Minitabs is not particularly good at dealing with large amounts of data or at carrying out cross-tabulations. Suppose for example you had carried out a survey where you had asked several hundred questions and you wanted to determine whether young people under the age of 25 answered these questions differently to those over the age of 26. This would be a very tedious process to carry out on Minitabs, but SPSSX (see below) could complete it in seconds.

References

Minitab Reference Manual (2nd edn) 1986. Minitab Incorporated, 3081 Enterprise Drive, State College, Pennsylvania 16801, USA.
Minitab Handbook (2nd edn) (by B. F. Ryan, B. L. Joiner & A. T. Ryan) 1985. PWS Publishers, Duxbury Press, Boston, USA.

SPSSX

SPSSX is the Statistical Package for Social Sciences, where X indicates that this is the tenth edition of the package.

SPSS is the most widely used statistical package for social science research. It is available for both microcomputers and mainframe computers. It is an excellent package for handling large amounts of data and can deal with thousands of variables on thousands of cases. Until recently it has only been available in batch mode, but there is a recent interactive edition. Because SPSSX is a quite complex system, it takes up a lot of storage space when used on a personal computer. It will carry out a wide variety of statistical manipulations and is good at summarising and presenting data graphically. With the current version it is not possible to calculate confidence intervals for parametric and non-parametric data, although this may change with future releases.

References

SPSSX Users' Guide. Marketing Department SPSS Inc. 3300444 North Michigan Avenue, Chicago, Illinois 60611, USA.
SPSSX Introductory Statistics Guide (by M. J. Norusis) 1983. SPSS Inc., address as above.
    There are other SPSS manuals including *SPSSX Basics*, which is a simple introduction for new users. There is an advanced statistics guide and a guide

that deals with data management. Compared with many packages, the manuals are reasonably easy to understand, although there are many terms that are not adequately defined and many procedures that are not clearly explained. It seems almost universal that people who design and write computer programs are unable to write about them in a way that is easily accessible to a general audience.

SPSSX is a very comprehensive system with a wide range of tests available. The manual runs to 806 pages of densely printed A4.

BMDP

BMDP stands for Biomedical Data Processing. This package comes from the University of California (UCLA). It is a powerful statistical program but is not as good as SPSSX at dealing with large quantities of data. However, it can perform several types of analysis that are not available on SPSSX. It is not very user-friendly and the 725-page manual is quite difficult to follow. The introduction to the manual suggests that the package has been designed for new and inexperienced users, as well as more experienced researchers. I think this statement should be treated with extreme caution.

Reference

BMDP Statistical Software (1981 edn) (by W. J. Dickson). University of California Press Limited, London, England.

Genstat

This is probably the most powerful statistical package currently available. It has really been written by statisticians for statisticians. It is almost indecipherable to a general user and I would not recommend its use at all.

Glim

Glim stands for Generalised Linear Interactive Modelling. It is a subset of the Genstat program particularly suitable for the analysis of survival times. The manual is virtually incomprehensible to a non-statistician and it is not suitable for beginners to research.

SAS

This is a statistical package particularly orientated towards IBM computers. Again, it is not a particularly easy package to use and I would not recommend it for a beginner.

Conclusions

This has been only a very brief introduction to the use of computers and the only way to learn is to sit down at a keyboard and practise. As well as producing statistical analyses, computers can help you in other ways. There are some very sophisticated graphics packages now available which will allow you to display your data in many different ways. Once you have entered your data on to a mainframe computer you can store it safely and keep it for many years. Most mainframe systems have an archiving storage facility to allow you to do this. You can also move your data around the country. There is a network called JANet (Joint Academic Network) which links Edinburgh, Newcastle, Cambridge, Manchester, Bristol, Exeter, Southampton, Oxford and London universities. There are gateways from this network to Europe and to America, so you can take your data with you if you move or even if you emigrate. At present, the main source for further information on using computers for statistical analysis are the statistical program manuals themselves, and I do not know of any book which sets down the principles in a simple way for the first-time user. As already mentioned, it is unfortunate that many of these manuals assume a great deal of prior knowledge about computing and statistics. If you are going to use computers on a regular basis, then it is best that you use one statistical package and try to become familiar with that and then ask for help if you need to use other packages. Many university departments run regular computing courses aimed at learning a specific package such as SPSSX or Minitabs, and it is worth inquiring at your nearest department of computer science about these.

Glossary

Blind

Double blind An experimental procedure, used particularly in drug trials, to guard against experimenter bias. It is arranged that neither the subjects nor the person gathering the data are aware which treatments are being given to which subjects.

Single blind This is where only one party (investigator or subject) is unaware as to which treatment group the subject belongs.

Triple blind This term is sometimes used to refer to studies where the patient, the rater, and the organiser of the study are all blind to the patient's group, so that all blood tests and data analysis are done on a blind basis. It can also apply to those (few) occasions when, in a double-blind assessment, neither party is aware that formal comparison is being made.

Blindness is also desirable in many other research designs. For example, in twin studies interviewers should not know whether they are interviewing a monozygotic or dizygotic twin.

Confidence interval An estimation of the limits within which a true finding or difference is likely to lie. This is usually expressed as a percentage. Thus a 95% confidence interval (or limit) is likely to contain the correct value of the finding 19 times out of 20 on average. Confidence intervals are now often preferred in the presentation of results because they reveal differences better than conventional tests of statistical significance.

Control group A group of subjects who are as similar to the experimental group as possible, with the exception of the variable(s) under study.

Historical controls The use of previously collected data for comparison with current data.

Concurrent controls This is where the control and experimental groups are collected at the same time, usually being randomly allocated from one sample.

Correlation A measure of the linear association between two continuous variables.

Experimenter bias   If a person conducting an experiment knows the experimental hypothesis, there is always some danger that he/she may unconsciously influence the results, in order to confirm the hypothesis.

Forced-choice technique   This is a technique introduced into attitude measurement to combat the tendency for the respondent to present him/herself in an over-favourable light. Items take the form of two or more statements, all of equal social desirability.

Halo effect   This is an effect which occurs when somebody making a judgement allows his/her general attitude to influence the answers to the particular items, as when the prettiest girl is also rated the most intelligent and the most sociable. In other words, she is being rated on a single concept, even though three separate answers are being produced.

Hawthorne effect   This is the unwitting introduction of extraneous variables through the social interaction of human experimenters and human subjects. This can grossly bias the results.

Hypothesis   An hypothesis is a conjecture about the relationship between two or more concepts. Hypotheses may be general assertions (e.g. man is innately aggressive), which are untestable in principle because of the imprecision of their concepts, or they may be more specific and narrow, and thus testable in principle if the concepts can be empirically interpreted (e.g. men with an extra chromosome will be more likely to commit violent crimes than men without an extra chromosome).

Null hypothesis   Before any hypothesis is tested statistically, it is always stated in the form of a null hypothesis, that is, that the test will reveal no differences between the groups being tested, no relationship between the variables of interest, etc.

Incidence   The number of episodes of an event (e.g. illness) or of individuals experiencing an event (e.g. becoming ill) beginning within a specified period of time. Thus annual incidence sets this period as one year.

Null hypothesis   The hypothesis that there is in reality no difference (or no degree of association) between two or more sets of data.

Pilot study   This is a small-scale, preliminary study undertaken to test the feasibility of the proposed research and to prove the procedures and methods of measurement.

Point prevalence   The number of episodes of an event (e.g. illness) or of individuals experiencing an event (e.g. becoming ill) existing at a specified point in time.

Power   (of a statistical test)   A measure of the likelihood of the test to reject the null hypothesis when the null hypothesis is incorrect (also see type II error).

Power function   The confidence level with which an investigator can claim that a defined benefit has not been overlooked. (In practice 80% power is a common aim.)

Prevalence   The number of episodes of an event (e.g. illness) or of individuals experiencing an event (e.g. becoming ill) existing within a specified time period (c.f. incidence).

Quota sampling   In this technique the population being sampled is divided, *before* sampling, into subgroups (e.g. social class), and the interviewers have to find a quota of people from each subgroup, so that the subgroups are in the same proportion in the sample as they are in the population.

Random allocation   People are allocated randomly to different groups and experiments, so that it is purely a matter of chance which person ends up in which group. The aim is to make the various groups comparable on all factors, except the independent variable, which can then be assigned by the researcher.

Rates   (e.g. hospital admission, mortality, incidence, prevalence)   The number of subjects affected expressed as a proportion of those at risk. These are usually expressed as numbers per population expressed as a power of 10 (e.g. 100, 1000, 100 000).

Rating scale   A scale in which any characteristic or rating is scored numerically. Such scales usually have three or more possible scores for each characteristic measured. When the intervals between each of the scores are equal the scale is sometimes described as a Likert or interval scale; when the scores are discrete and easily separated the scale is a categorical one; and when the intervals are very many and consecutive intervals not clearly defined the scale is a continuous one. The extreme of a continuous scale is the visual analogue scale, in which the range of scores is represented as a continuous line which is completed by entering a mark across the line at the appropriate level of intensity.

Regression   A measure of the dependence of one variable on one or more other variables.

Reliability   The extent to which a test would give consistent results on being applied more than once to the same people under standard conditions.

Split-half method   The scores on a randomly chosen half of the test questions are correlated with the scores on the other half.

Cronbach's α   This is the mean value of all the possible split-half reliability coefficients. The above two are measures of internal consistency.

Test–retest reliability   This is where a correlation is obtained between scores on the test administered to the same people, but on separate occasions.

Alternate-form reliability   This is similar, except that the second form of the test is as nearly equivalent to the first as possible.

Inter-rater reliability   This refers to the extent to which two raters making the same series of judgements would get the same results.

Response bias   A systematic bias or set pervading someone's answers to a test.

Acquiescence response test   This is a tendency to answer positively to questions on a questionnaire, irrespective of their content.

Extreme responding   This is a tendency to select extreme alternatives to items in a test.

Social desirability   This is a response set in which one responds either consciously or unconsciously in such a way as to make a good impression.
Methods for combating response bias include lie scales, which consist of items in which one of the alternatives is too good to be true, and the use of a forced-choice technique.

Response rate   In a survey the response rate is a percentage of the sample chosen who actually participate. There is virtually always a proportion who refuse or who cannot be found. Although there are no hard and fast rules, 90% or above of the respondents would be considered a high response rate for most purposes: 70–80% might be considered as acceptable.

Sample   This is a group selected from a large population with the aim of yielding information about the population as a whole.

Sampling frame   This is a record or set of records which sets out and identifies the population from which a sample is to be drawn (e.g. the electoral roll, the list of patients in a general practice or a list of all local authority primary schools).

Scatter diagram   A graph showing the relationship between two characteristics in which each individual showing the characteristics is included as a point or dot.

Sequential designs   Treatment designs that use the results to determine the length of the study. If there is a large difference between treatments fewer patients are needed than if there is a small or negligible difference.

Statistical significance   An indication of the plausibility that data differences could have arisen by chance.

Stratification   This is the division of a research cohort into layers or strata, for example by sex or social class. This is so as to be able to draw a random sample from each layer and therefore increase the precision of the sample without having to increase its size.

Type I error   To commit a type I error is to reject the null hypothesis when it is true. The probability, designated α, of making a type I error is specified by the researcher before testing the hypothesis.

Type II error   To commit a type II error is to accept the null hypothesis when it is false. The probability, designated β, of making a type II error is specified by the researcher before testing the hypothesis. This type of error is particularly likely with small samples. The probability of making a type II error is normally greater than for a type I error.

Validity   Traditionally this is the extent to which a test or questionnaire (or any other operationalisation) is really measuring what the researcher intends it to measure. The modern emphasis is more on the extent to which the measure bears out the properties assigned to it by the theory in which it plays a part.

Face validity   This is the extent to which the test contains items which intuitively appear to be valid.

Concurrent validity   If it correlates well with other measures of the same concept, then the validity is concurrent.

Content validity   This is when it adequately samples the domain that it is supposed to measure.

Predictive validity   This is when it may be used to make accurate prediction of future performance.

Construct validity   This refers to the extent to which the test appears to conform to predictions about it from theory, or from other relevant observations.

Variables   Variables are constructs or events that are studied in research.

Independent variable   This is the condition which is manipulated or altered by the experimenter (e.g. giving a drug, altering a drug, giving ECT).

Dependent variable   This is a variable used to measure the effect of the independent variables, such as a rating-scale score, length of time in hospital, etc. Most studies use a number of dependent variables.

Confounding variable   This is any extraneous variable which may potentially have an effect on the dependent variable and which has not been controlled for. Normally one tries to reduce confounding variables by using matched control groups.

Controlled variable   This is a variable where the experimenter attempts to keep its influence constant (e.g. night sedation, amount of attention from nurses).

Uncontrolled variable   Many epidemiological studies deal with this sort of phenomena. This is a variable which is not manipulated or held constant by the experimenter, but an event which occurs and is then measured (e.g. life event, suicide attempt).

Index

Compiled by **STANLEY THORLEY**

Page references to figures and tables are set in italic type.